ASTONISH ME

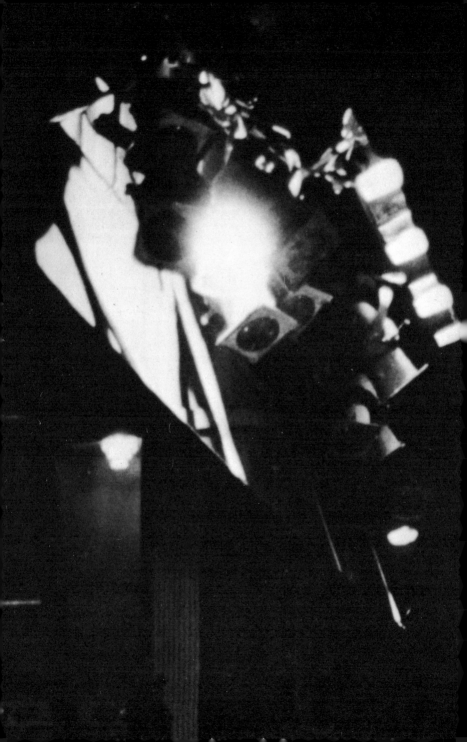

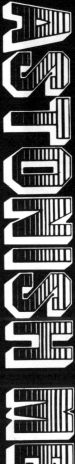

ASTONISH ME

Adventures in Contemporary Theater

JOHN LAHR

A RICHARD SEAVER BOOK

The Viking Press / *New York*

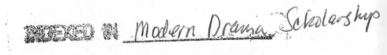 INDEXED IN *Modern Drama Scholarship*

To my mother, Mildred;
and once again to my beloved Anthea.

And in memory of Bert Lahr,
the most astonishing performer of them all.

Acknowledgments

Writing criticism, like any performance, is an act of discovery. Although promoted as a star turn, criticism is no solo enterprise. Any collection of my essays owes a debt to Fred Jordan of Grove Press, who first offered me the opportunity to speak my mind every month in *Evergreen Review*. Ross Wetzsteon, Ed Fancher, and Dan Wolf gave me a berth on *The Village Voice* and the freedom to write what I want when I want. Dick and Jeannette Seaver, my friends and editors, have believed in my approach to theater and given me the honor of being on the first list of Richard Seaver Books.

Anthea Lahr, my wife, has policed every word of these essays. Through her questions, criticism, and blue pencil, this book—and my writing in general—has been immeasurably improved.

Contents

PERFORMANCES

Illustrations

(Following page 182)

The Hippogriff—from *Orlando Furioso*

The Marine Bear—from *Orlando Furioso*

Soldiers fighting—from *Orlando Furioso*

The King and Queen fleeing from Varennes—from *1789*

Puppets—from *1789*

Perowne and Sadie in Perowne's room—from *AC/DC*

Snake strangling inquisitive tourist—from *Operation Sidewinder*

The Man Who Smiles and the Ringmaster—from *The Mutation Show*

The imprisoned speak—from *Terminal*

The Berrigans burning draft cards

Muhammad Ali in *Big Time Buck White*

Alice and the Sea Serpent—from *Alice in Wonderland*

PAGEANTS

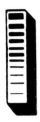

Orlando Furioso:
Theater as
"Contact" Sport

Habit is a great deadener.
—SAMUEL BECKETT

Orlando Furioso is great theater. Epic, gigantic, operatic, and outrageous—it is like walking into your most heroic dream awake. Performed in Italian by the Teatro Libero di Roma (a cast of sixty-three), its appearance in America is a major event at a time when theater must redefine itself if it is to survive in competition with other media.

Orlando Furioso breaks almost every rule of our conventional stage, and, bold enough to be simple, it is a profound experience. The event brings an audience back to an understanding of the primal ingredients of stagecraft: energy and astonishment. The tale is the familiar romantic picaresque quest: knights-errant and damsels in distress, wizards and wondrous accomplishments. Orlando dreams his beloved Angelica is in danger. He sets out to find her. In this stage event, the audience, too, becomes a community of seekers. *Orlando* is based on Ariosto's epic poem (1516); but the picaresque tradition is not arcane, it survives in American Westerns. Action, not refinement of thought, is the order of the day; the values of loyalty, chastity, and courage are tested by men of action in heroic battles and miraculous escapes. Swirling through the standing audience on platforms reminiscent of the medieval *platea,* the actors tower above the people in the audience and hurtle dangerously between them. Instead of one plot and one platform, there are many. The audience cannot "sit still" or absorb the "through-line" of action. The density of the event forces them to open themselves up to the total theatrical experience. Entering *Orlando* is like comprehending a Pollock painting; where the meaning *is* the action. The audience must accept it, find a place to begin, then follow the energy. No one will see the same thing; no action is repeatable. Watching *Orlando* is like gazing into cut glass—a refraction of brilliant contours. Thought, theme, and texture come after the experience: *Orlando* sweeps an audience up in the precipitous thrill, size, and mystery of the moment. Delight disregards temporary confusion: the audience learns to adapt to the rules of the event. They are players in a game they find irresistible. Theater becomes sport; and in one of those rare festival moments of which only the stage is capable, the theater becomes an exemplary action, bringing people together in a new way; instructing the imagination while pleasing it; pointing highly successful and professional techniques toward new theater while rediscovering a continuity with dramatic and literary traditions of the past.

No theater event has dealt so boldly and surely with the problems of conventional theater and audience as *Orlando Furioso*; and no production of such indubitable excellence has met with such tepid, misinformed, and fossilized response from New York's daily drama critics. *Orlando Furioso* forces not only a re-examination of the essential equations of theater, but also the nature of daily criticism, which responds more easily to formula than to original and authentic stage experience. Audiences, not critics, kept *Orlando* alive in America. This is a people's theater: a humanizing initiation into emotion and relation that our technological society limits. In discovering the jolting exchange of energy between actor and audience, the sensual and kinetic thrill of bodies moving in space, audiences have glimpsed what theater can be: not an exercise in evasion, but confrontation; not cultural shadowboxing, but an active contest of wills. *Orlando* changes us and our ideas of theater.

I

Theater consists of bodies in space, and space itself is dramatic. American audiences are conditioned to the flatness of the proscenium picture stage and the assumptions of its one-point perspective. Look at any conventional theater when the house is empty. Each seat is pointed toward the stage: numbered, raked, isolated by armrests from the next viewer. Like the majority of the plays these theaters house, the message built into the architecture is "sit tight." Only one fifth of this overdecorated room we call a theater is being used for "play." The audience is compartmentalized. There is a ghostly, static uniformity in the architecture— just as the one-point perspective attempts to make space itself *static* for the viewer. Significantly, the environment on stage is called "a set." Everyone is supposed to see the same thing (of course, those who pay more get closer to the action). But, as anthropologist Edward T. Hall has pointed out:

> To hold space static and organize the elements of space so as to be viewed from a single point [is] in reality to treat three-dimensional space in a *two-dimensional manner.* Because the stationary *eye* flattens things out beyond sixteen feet, it is possible to do just this—treat space optically. The *trompe l'œil* so popular in the Renaissance and succeeding periods epitomizes the visual space as seen from a single point.[1] *

The proscenium and the raked seats separate the audience from the performers. In a culture which likes to keep things "normal," which tranquilizes itself to avoid passion and puts its "disturbed" out of sight, emotion and action are kept at a safe, unbreachable distance. *Orlando Furioso*, on the other hand, exploits the drama of actor and audience existing in a fluid, highly charged space. This is a festival of spirit. Nothing holds its shape; even the play's proscenium settings move out into the audience. Here, no space is "dead"; no experience so distant and passive that it can be discussed in the literary, linear vocabulary of proscenium theater, which defines its action in terms of "plot points," "through-lines," gestures which "read" to an audience. The magic of *Orlando* is the choreography of performance. There is no *trompe l'œil*: artifice is the only reality. All the machinery of make-believe is clearly visible. Stagehands crouch to

* These numbers refer to notes to be found on page 257.

propel the platforms through the crowds and open trap doors; actors hide behind revolves before making "miraculous" appearances. The acceptance of the artificiality of the event makes the impact of each image more wonderful and immediate. The shock brought conditioned reflexes from many of the old-guard play reviewers. Richard Watts of the *New York Post* wrote, "Personally I would be more content to sit in the 15th row far on one side at a play on a stage." Although his seats are better, this is precisely what he has been doing for half a century.

Orlando dramatizes the liberating forces of three-dimensional space: the tactile pleasure and danger of inhabiting it. The audience is not frozen into one posture or perspective. They can examine performances with microscopic detail, or watch the prehistoric Hippogriff—a colossal hybrid with wings of a flying fish and the head of a griffin—as it soars high above the heads of the crowd and swings closer toward them. To see it on the wing is to remember Icarus's dream and why he imagined it. The event takes place in a space the size of a football field, with two mammoth ornamental curtains—one russet, the other a Tintoretto-blue sky—humorous "boundaries" of the event. These are the conventional curtains of the proscenium stage, but nothing that comes out from underneath them will be safe, static, or predictable. *Orlando* is a difficult but important ritual for a culture so numb to and careless about its environment that it either destroys its natural surroundings or passes through them in prefabricated insulation. The only way to evade the dramatic environment is by completely dropping out of the action and excitement to bleachers on the side of the arena. Here, there is a conventional distance between spectators and spectacle, but no meaning for the viewer. *Orlando*

Furioso's energy is so luminous that people are lured out of their fatigue and apprehension back into the vortex of this playground.

The entire playing area is tense in the atmosphere of the unexpected. Spaces expand and contract, so do the public's position in them. Platforms divide and combine as fluidly as raindrops. Nothing can be taken for granted; the environment is not "set." At one moment, the audience can be in the center of the arena, clustered comfortably around an ecstatic love duet between Bradamante (a maiden disguised as a man) and her long-lost lover, Ruggiero; in the next, they can be skittering like waterbugs for the safety of the sidelines as six twenty-foot horses bear down on them in battle. The environment becomes a test: a puzzle in which stamina, courage, ingenuity, curiosity, help solve the theatrical riddle. The audience must be quick, agile, inventive. The whole body is at play. Running for safety, dodging platforms and wooden-sword fights, finding the action— theater becomes a "contact" sport in which the audience and actor battle for space and each other's energy. The competition is not only between the actors for the audience's attention, but between the spectators themselves for new sights and sounds amidst the incredible variety and detail of the production. The mercurial nature of the environment emphasizes the glorious transience of performance. The audience must savor each moment, or miss it.

II

"Theater as a social happening may have possibilities."[2] Clive Barnes's statement is indicative of how far American theater has strayed from its primal impulse. Theater is nothing if not a social happening. Like the medieval festivals, *Orlando* emphasizes community, not isolation. Television and film reinforce man's isolation; theater—at its best —emphasizes human interdependence. Jacques Ellul has written:

> Television, because of its power of fascination and its capacity of visual and auditory penetration, is probably the technical instrument which is most destructive of personality and of human relations. What man seeks is evidently an absolute distraction, a total obliviousness of himself and his problems and the simultaneous fusion of his consciousness with an omnipresent technical diversion.[3]

In *Orlando*, the spectator is made *self*-aware, defining himself in the moment and not obliterating it. The audience helps one another. The crowd (about 1000 a night) begins by attempting to follow the action from the printed scenario. But words are not enough. Action is the only *fact*. (The program reads: "*Orlando Furioso* is mostly about some French and Saracen warriors who chase women when they are not chasing each other.") People begin to talk to one another: pointing out new scenes, identifying characters, pulling each other away from fast-moving platforms, guiding people to positions from which to see the next astonishing spectacle. Information and space are shared. The distance between people, enforced by a proscenium theater, is broken down. W. H. Auden wrote of the psychic no-trespassing sign which is an attitude reflected and implied in our conventional theater:

> Some thirty inches from my nose
> The frontier of my Person goes
> And all the untilled air between

Is private pagus or demesne.
Stranger, unless with bedroom eyes
I beckon you to fraternize,
Beware of rudely crossing it:
I have no gun, but I can spit.

—"Prologue: The Birth of Architecture"

The amount of distance we put between events and ourselves is a cultural bias. Anglo-Saxon individualism is offended by proximity. But the slap and tickle of actor and audience in *Orlando* is a seduction of such grace and good humor that audiences are bound together in a common, joyful endeavor.

Free from the conventional restrictions implicit in "taking a seat" (e.g., to "keep still" and "be quiet"), the audience re-creates a sense of its own freedom and power. *Orlando* encourages and can absorb vocal emotions. The audience bravos the spectacle when it takes outrageous melodramatic turns: the *distraite* Angelica, sighing with hands on breast, as, forlornly, she passes her mounted swain; the flamboyant good fairy, Melissa, who enters through a trap door holding a magic ring for Bradamante in distress, pointing heavenward with one hand, encouraging applause with the other. The spectators hiss the green-faced wizard, Atlante; or the conniving Monk who makes no secret of the sacrifice he wants the prostrate Angelica to make. Much against their usual habit of theatergoing, spectators find themselves momentarily pushing the platforms or reaching out to touch an actor in the maze. The energy breeds engagement, not escape.

Most American theater, like the culture it serves, is an exercise in internalization of feeling. *Orlando Furioso* encourages emotional "initiative."[4] There is no programed time or place to display emotion; there is no single emotion which is the only response at a given moment. But Americans are nervous with people who "make scenes"; they don't like to make a "show" of emotions. Our society emphasizes—because of its Puritan origins and the continual abrasion of its technological ethos—"keeping cool." In America, everything from television to tranquilizers, bureaucracy to business, reinforces the internalizing of response. The actors of Teatro Libero felt this cultural timidity. "Why they take hand away?" asked one actress who placed the hand of a spectator firmly on her breast, only to have it pulled away. The process of such full and authentic participation is a healthy antidote to a society with deep internal controls, so fearful and confused about emotion. Sociologist Philip Slater has observed:

> Where internalization is high there is often a feeling that the controls themselves are out of control—that emotion cannot be expressed when the individual would like to express it. Life is muted, experience filtered, emotion anesthetized, affective discharge incomplete. Efforts to shake free from this hypertrophied control system include not only drugs and sensation-retrieval techniques such as those developed at the Esalen Institute in California, but also confused attempts to re-establish external systems of direction and control—the vogue currently enjoyed by astrology is an expression of this.[5]

In astounding its audiences, *Orlando Furioso* allows them to locate resources of emotion and energy in themselves. The theater fills the viewer with the pulse of active life. The spectators are genuinely at play; and this is an act of renewal.

III

Performing is a kind of ecstasy, an act so inspired and ir-rational that—at its extremes—it can seem vulgar, lunatic, and dangerous. America knew this flamboyant explosion of passion in its stage clowns and wasn't afraid of their mad-ness. Our language for their cavorting indicates how far beyond the reasoning intellect performance could go: "wild," "zany," "insane," "mayhem," "bedlam," "lunacy." But now we are a fearful society, increasingly cut off from our bodies. Our obsession with control is reinforced by the images of ourselves we incessantly observe and hold as ideal models. Actors, like audiences, seem to be ossified. Even our comedians are called "stand-up," indicating, sadly, how lit-tle movement remains in their craft. Television and film continually tone down gesture so that it won't appear gro-tesque under the scrutiny of the close-up. Performing, the spectacle of chameleon energy, has become a frozen tab-leau. But the essential thrill of performance is seeing bodies extend and transform themselves before our eyes. Perform-ing is "showing off" (an emotion to an audience). *The New York Times'* second-stringer Mel Gussow criticized *Orlando Furioso* for being "a spectacle which made a public spectacle of itself." This was meant to be derogatory; but, in the finest clowning tradition, no words could prove its essential purity with more clarity. Performing is energy calling attention to itself, drawing people close to its high voltage. Young audi-ences appreciate the energy of Mick Jagger and Jimi Hen-drix. But rock is shallow, makeshift theater compared to what the stage can provide. Yet rarely does our modern the-ater offer a chance to experience such an authentic spectacle of performing. The language of our approval ("I eat it up," "I crave it," "I can't get enough," "I lap it up") indicates how audiences long to swallow the event, to literally take it in. *Orlando Furioso* makes this performing energy accessible and unforgettable.

Orlando Furioso is essentially street theater; and this is a viable format—with its bravado and parody—for the operatic exaggeration of its actors. Gestures must be broad in order to be seen; emotions must be grandiose in a play imitating heroic legend. Performing is outrageous; what is real is not the outer façade of action, but the inner emotion driving the body to such extremes. Clive Barnes referred to the acting in *Orlando* as "amateurish." His confusion about the high quality of the Libero's performance comes from not really knowing the dynamics of street theater and the broadness such an environment demands. Professionalism is relative. The finest Broadway actress, if put in a street-theater situation, where audiences are talking, where she has to vie for attention, might not be "professional." The performing in *Orlando* is explosive, not contained.

Spoken in Italian, the acting in *Orlando* makes audiences aware of the surprise of language and its relation to gesture. Emanating not from the mouth but through the body, the word is not the first expression of the performer. The word is the final incarnation of a physical idea. Everything spoken in Italian has to be pushed out into the world through gestures. Movement and speech exist in gorgeous counterpoint. There is never a moment when a performer's intention or his meaning is unclear. The audience reads the signals of the body and the voice. Like burlesque, *Orlando Furioso* creates an atmosphere where the actors can pull out all the stops. They are in their own emotional orbit: mugging, declaiming, dancing, pratfalling. Olimpia's words rise into operatic arias. Voices whisper and shout, rumble and proclaim. The heroic sound envelops the audience. Actors expressing "tragic loss" reach out at first to characters, then to the audience. The illusion works brilliantly. Spectators become actors. At one performance, an actor held a woman's hand, hugging it against his face in grief. The platform was being pushed away as if a chapter of Ariosto's epic had been closed and a new one about to begin. The spectator did not let go of the actor's hand. She moved with him as the platform receded. The actor kept talking to her even out of earshot of the rest of the audience, who had turned to look elsewhere for new action. The Libero actors perform this spectacle with immense conviction, adding both humor and credibility to its mythic proportions.

Fingers, eyes, lips, torso exist at a sensual proximity that no theatergoer has ever been allowed to observe on the proscenium stage. The actors are athletes and acrobats—jumping from one platform to another, wrestling, running. They are also mimes, creating the illusion of unseen worlds through gesture. Orlando battles the Marine Bear—a mammoth vertebrate that rolls out from behind the curtain and threatens to swallow Olimpia. Running full tilt and wielding an anchor, the beast suddenly splits to encase Orlando and spin him about. The moment is astounding. After Orlando hacks at the beast, he swims away. Actors carry him, kicking and stroking, back to the safety of his platform. The playfulness of the idea and its execution is typical of the carnival spirit *Orlando* evokes. The performer is once again returned to the role of delightful chameleon, appearing unexpectedly pushing a platform one minute, the center of attention in a new costume the next. He has many disguises and poses. He is playing a wondrous shell game with the audience and himself.

IV

Theater must reclaim space as a playground. Theater must usher us into the unknown, offering us an extraordinary and unique world as an alternative to our daily lives. *Orlando Furioso* does this. *The New York Times* called the show "ridiculous." It is right. Orlando whirls around an audience with the inspired ridiculousness of a Keaton, a Marx brother, or a Lahr. Theirs was not a theater of statement, but of experience. So is *Orlando*. The *brio* of the performing, the genius of the manipulation of space (staged by Luca Ronconi) makes participating in the joy of the event its true relevance. In a nation of watchers, the theater must remind us of our power to play and recreate.

Orlando is not spectacle for its own sake. There is an intellectual integrity behind the production's epic size and the atmosphere of astonishment. The endless ritual battles, the disguises and magical escapes, have a repetition and fun in performance which make their comment on the idealization of heroic legend. The ideals of loyalty, romantic love, military courage, are not things we can respect in our betrayed, jaded, modern imaginations. Mystery has been sacrificed to technology; language replaced by bureaucratic rhetoric. Renaissance folklore—its cultish violence parading as valor, its alabaster virtue—is as preposterous and artificial as the action in *Orlando*.

The production is not simply high camp (although when one maiden, Alcina, enters in a gold mask and a Degas tutu accompanied by an attendant blowing bubbles, the joke almost gives itself away). At the end of the play, a labyrinth is pushed out into the central playing area. The spectators move through it. Around them are cages—now madhouses—where the characters re-enact the play's events. The moment is stunning. The visual image sardonically brings the playfulness into modern focus, revealing the characters trapped in the madness of their "tragic" rhetoric and the melodramatic "logic" of their actions. Legends have come off the page and are now exhibited like fairground curiosities. The audience strolls from cage to cage: staring, making faces, testing the energy of each performer as he recounts his tales with obsessed passion.

As Astolfo rides the Hippogriff to the moon, the lights dim to focus on him. The actors slip away in the darkness. When the lights come up, what is left of the fabulous event is the audience groping through the chicken-wire labyrinth. *They* are in the cages. *They* are looking at each other: actors in their own drama. Their gestures, their clothes, have their own extravagance and exaggeration; their relationships are as melodramatic, idealized, and perhaps as hollow as the world they've enjoyed. They look in vain for signs of the monumental energy and artifice. They see only themselves.

In the white light, dwarfed in the massive space, the reason for dreaming and playing is made clear. We are such small, timorous souls with such gargantuan appetites. What is there for us but the imagined strength and comforting evasion of myth?

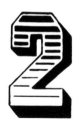

The Theater
of Sports

The human being is delivered helpless, in
respect to life's most important and trivial
affairs, to a power (technology) which is in no
sense under his control. For there can be no
question today of man's controlling the milk
he drinks or the bread he eats, any more than
of his controlling his government.

   —JACQUES ELLUL, *The Technological Society*

Take me out to the ball game,
Take me out to the park.
Buy me some peanuts and Cracker Jack,
I don't care if I never get back. . . .

   —Old baseball song

Games are a means, through make-believe, of coping with
the world. So is theater. But as the opportunity for physical

prowess and uncomplicated, noble victory is denied mechanized man, the spectacle of sport has assumed a potency
and ritual importance in America that most theater has
lost. Sports have become a twentieth-century obsession, the
nation's grand distraction—incorporating a tableau of
affluence and energy once reserved for the Broadway musical into the larger ambitions of a highly industrial state.
Formal, controlled, efficiently organized, the modern spectacles reflect the technological thrust of this century. They
offer not only escape but confirmation, adjusting the public
to the violence and inequities of the system. Theater, emphasizing immediacy, emotional depth, psychic and social
change, is reminiscent of a humanity being eroded by
urban living. Spectacle is more comfortable and reassuring.
It asks no questions of the viewer but provides the thrill of
external action.

The sports spectacle has become America's right-wing
theater, affirming the *status quo* by making those processes
which emasculate man palatable in "play." Spectacle is an
important barometer of an age. Each type of spectacle has
evolved with the demands of contemporary society, reflect-
ing and influencing its view of the world.

I

Medieval pageants were a concrete expression of the living faith. They brought the teachings of the Church off the
cathedral walls and into the town square. The floats, which
squeaked under the weight of peasant angels, devils, and
biblical heroes, were preceded at each station by the blare
of trumpets and the hoots of an obstreperous crowd. The
spectacles were an escape and an educational device, as

well as a means of keeping the feudal population obedient to the Church. Spectacle was a community activity. In the town of Wakefield, which produced the memorable cycle of mystery plays, records show that two hundred and forty parts were filled from a town of approximately five hundred and sixty people. The guilds competed in building floats. The actors, miming the drama of Heaven and Hell which surrounded their lives, often played roles parallel to their position in the town pecking order.

Although the pageants were referred to as "mystery" plays, there was no mystery for the medieval audience to whom the stories were a familiar affirmation of the Church's truth. With pulleys to suspend angels and trapdoors to dispatch devils, the medieval multiple set reinforced the hierarchical view of man's place in the divine scheme. The process of man's life was not as important as the reassuring iconography that surrounded it. The groupings, gestures, symbols in spectacle had an orthodoxy that the words did not. The spectacle incarnated the medieval mentality, communicating in sculptural, vivid images to nonliterate medieval minds. The simple images made profound sense of a confusing world. The people witnessing the spectacle were intimately involved with those performing it. They were seeing the divine in themselves and themselves in the divine. The effect was to create a political as well as spiritual unity: "The crowd assembled for the great festivals felt itself to be a living whole, and became the mystical body of Christ, its soul passing into his Soul." [1]

While spoken sermons were few in the Middle Ages (a thirteenth-century papal decree commanded at least four a year), spectacle was used by radical priests like Saint Francis of Assisi (who went among the people and made a "spectacle of himself ") to dramatize the necessity of a saintly life and the onus of sin. Saint Francis's attempt to embrace the formula of spectacle for individual drama is described by Erich Auerbach:

> He forced his inner impulse into outer forms; his being and his life became public events; from the day when, to signify his relinquishment of things of the world, he gave back his clothes to his upbraiding father, down to the day when, dying, he had himself laid naked on the naked earth so that in his last hour, when the archfiend might still rage, he could fight naked with the naked enemy.[2]

Saint Francis confronted his audience with immediate images. After a night of gluttony, he had himself dragged through the town with a rope around his neck while he confessed. The spectacle matched the pageants in clarity and scenic force. It demanded imitation and participation by the community. Saint Francis used the contemporary sense of the world to captivate an audience.

In Elizabethan England spectacle was also a means of community control. The seasonal celebrations were organized anarchy intended to take the head off the frustration and violence of a stratified society. The Lord and Lady of Misrule mocked the Lords and Ladies of the Manor by mimicking and exaggerating their power. A Puritan observer described a typical May game:

> They have twenty or forty yoke of oxen, every oxe having a sweet nosegay of flowers on the tip of his horns, and these oxen draw home this Maypole which is covered all over with flowers and herbs, bound round about with strings, from the top to the bottom . . . with two or three hundred men, women and children following it with great devotion. And thus being reared up with handkerchiefs and flags . . .

they strew the ground about, bind green boughs about it, set up summer halls, bowers and arbors hard by it. And then they fall to dance about it, like as the heathen people did at the dedication of Idols. . . .[3]

Trespassing beyond the allotted festival period could bring severe penalties. But, once begun, the momentum of spectacle was sometimes hard to stop. In *Henry IV* (Part 1), Prince Hal criticizes Falstaff, the archetypal Lord of Misrule, who forgets the boundaries of spectacle:

If all the year were playing holidays,
To sport would be as tedious as to work;
But when they seldom come, they wish'd for come. . . .
—(I, ii, 217–219)

As C. L. Barber writes in *Shakespeare's Festive Comedy*, the anarchy allowed the mock lord to enjoy "building up his dignity, and also exploding it by exaggeration, while his followers both relish his bombast as a fleer at proper authority and also enjoy turning on him and insulting his majesty . . . the game at once appropriates and annihilates the mana of authority." [4] These popular spectacles fed theater, especially Shakespeare's comedies. Shakespeare transported this "midsummer madness" to the stage, not merely by adopting its sights and sounds, but by applying the festival process of release and clarification through playing. In Shakespeare's comedies the characters move into a safe, festival world (Arden, Oberon's Wood, Olivia's house), where identities are tested and explored. Shakespeare's characters often game at the world in order to discover it, while remaining outside its passions. Viola says of Feste in *Twelfth Night*:

This fellow is wise enough to play the fool;
And to do that well craves a kind of wit:
He must observe the mood on whom he jests,
The quality of persons, and the time. . . .

—(III, i, 59–62)

Festivals dramatized identity; people found out about the world by playing at it. In *As You Like It*, Rosalind escapes the chaos of the court, discovers the "liberty" of Arden, and finally returns to the real world. She is now socially and psychically whole. The play parallels the process of Elizabethan spectacle, a game which clarifies the actual experience.

Feste's final song in *Twelfth Night*—"The rain that raineth every day"—emphasizes the stark reality which makes it necessary to play but also to realize the limitation of the spectacle. The paradox is built into the sadness of Feste's chronicle of his life:

But when I came to man's estate,
    With hey, ho, the wind and the rain,
'Gainst knaves and thieves men shut their gate,
    For the rain it raineth every day.

—(V, i, 387–390)

Twelfth Night's popularity rests with Shakespeare's ability to harness the frenzy of folk spectacle to more responsible ends.

II

The pressure of technology molds the form of modern spectacle. Games admit a mechanized sense of time; they stress a closed system of rules and moves. Spectacle, before the development of technique, was eccentric. The modern spectacle has become national through the television set. Now the most popular modern spectator sports (baseball, football) are not the ones which Americans play most (golf, bowling). Football and baseball can be enjoyed in statistics as well as on the field. They have a fictional appeal in a society whose organization fractures work and puts a premium on efficiency rather than imagination. Sports recast man in a heroic mold. They are important for creating a sense of well-being in troubled times.

As the primal sources of man's identity are strangled by technology, as his primacy and his relation to the land are minimized, his fanaticism toward sports increases. Technology is both an oppressor and a reason for hope. The modern American games try to palliate this paradox. But the spectacles which set out to be diversion end up as cultural anesthesia. From childhood, the American male is steeped in the rules and lore of the games which imbue control, team play, and moral value. Life is equated with sports; the body (especially in football) aspires to become the machine which has replaced it in the real world. The spectacles institutionalize conformity and obedience, laying the groundwork for totalitarian response. The stress on toughness and violent victory ("slaughter," "kill," "pound," "ream," "cream," "mutilate") indicates a primitive militarism. Football vernacular betrays the game's martial fantasy. The quarterback, "a field general," throws "bullet" passes or "the long bomb." The "scouts" help him analyze the "defense," whose tactics include "blitzing" and "submarining."

Technicized sport was first developed in the United States, the most conformist of all countries, and . . . it was then developed as a matter of course by the dictatorships, Fascist, Nazi, and Communist, to the point that it became an indispensable constituent element of totalitarian regimes.[5]

Sport allows the culture—so conscious of the failures of its value structure—to be absorbed in a fantasy of victory where pluck 'n' luck pay off. The game quickly takes on real-life overtones. Talking about the naturalness of tackling in football, Vince Lombardi once observed, "If a man is running down the street with everything you own, you won't let him get away. That's tackling." Football dramatizes not only possession, but survival. It is not surprising that a society motivated and eroded by an ethic of individual enterprise should create a spectacle of Darwinian struggle. The former New York Jet All-Pro end George Sauer has defined this obsession:

> There is unqualified effort to overcome and rise above the other man, and to be Number One is the ultimate objective. As the fittest are in the process of surviving, almost any means may be employed for their aggrandizement. . . .
>
> One of the most admired traits in football is aggressiveness toward the opponent. . . . One mandatory quality for football players is to withstand intimidation. Rules are by no means inviolable, and intentional transgressions are deemed integral to the pursuance of the end: the survival of the fittest. . . . The opponent is judged by the superficial criterion of uniform color. This serves to determine the ethicality—or its absence—of the opponent's particular actions, and what may be condemned in him may be justified in oneself. To attempt to generate hate for an opponent is considered conducive to the realizing of the end of establishing superiority. . . . It seems that physical degradation is an ingrained feature of football.

In both football and baseball, black men have only recently figured prominently. Although Jackie Robinson broke baseball's color barrier in 1947, a decade later there were only twelve Negro ballplayers in the National League, and, as late as 1960, there were as few as six blacks in the American League![6] Even now, although the percentage of black players is higher, the games still accustom spectators to the black man's peripheral role in society. As with any theatrical production, grouping carries its special moral overtones. In baseball, the majority of black players are outside the center of activity, supporting a structure while rarely being central to it. They interact less frequently. Comparing race and position in major-league baseball, sociologists discovered data which confirmed the unstated bias of the game. In 1967, blacks filled only 19 of 113 infield positions.

| Playing Position | Both Leagues[7] | |
	White	Black
Catcher	27	1
Shortstop	17	1
First base	18	7
Second base	16	4
Third base	16	6
Outfield	38	36

The same pattern recurs in football. Blacks rarely occupy pivotal positions (on offense: center, guards, and quarterback; on defense, the linebackers).

Football dramatizes blacks as less visible, often high-stepping functionaries. Our fantasy systems act out the nation's ingrained racism. In play, as in life, the people who call the signals are white. It is their rules, their dream, and their

POSITION OCCUPANCY WITH OFFENSIVE TEAMS[8]

Playing Position	Both Leagues	
	White	Black
Pivotal Positions		
Center	26	0
Quarterback	25	1
Right guard	24	2
Left guard	25	1
Right tackle	21	5
Left tackle	19	7
Tight end	20	6
Split end	18	8
Fullback	15	11
Halfback	10	16
Flankerback	17	9

POSITION OCCUPANCY WITH DEFENSIVE TEAMS[9]

Playing Position	Both Leagues	
	White	Black
Pivotal Positions		
Middle linebacker	24	2
Right linebacker	25	1
Left linebacker	23	3
Right end	18	8
Right tackle	20	6
Left tackle	17	9
Left end	19	7
Right safety	17	9
Left safety	17	9
Right cornerback	8	18
Left cornerback	4	22

need to forget which elevate the game to its cultural importance.

Sports spectacles also feed a larger psychic yearning: the illusion of primitive power, now lost to the machine. As Lionel Tiger points out in *Men in Groups* (Random House, 1969), sports allow the spectator to rediscover his identity through "hunter-aggressive endeavors." The team names dramatize the spectators' wish-fulfillment: animals in the chase (Falcons, Tigers, Cubs, Bears, Hawks, Broncos), or heroic figures of power and bravery (Buffalo Bills, Giants, Vikings, Warriors, Braves).

Baseball is a spectacle of America's early industrialization, a game of "one thing at a time, fixed positions, and visibly delegated specialist jobs." [10] Football is the daydream of a passive, computerized society, melding violence with elaborate efficiency. They are both epic struggles which have their real-life consummation in the astronauts, the game of the technological present. The space game takes its place as a popular spectacle, exhibiting the national fascination with teamwork and hardware which rationalizes and sublimates the social ulcer. With astronautics, the machine becomes the hero of the spectacle, assuming the mythic power once invested in man. The space program is named "Apollo"; the moonship has the imperial, predatory title of "Eagle"; and even the NASA satellites are called "Mariner," an image reminiscent of Viking journeys into uncharted waters, also a test of selfhood. The goal of these crew-cut sons of technology is nothing less than perfection—"zero defects."

All these spectacles emphasize the American articles of faith: accomplishment, production, bravery, and goodness. In breaking in an audience to its technological environment, modern spectacle answers to the demands of the people. As individuality decreases in America, sports turn human beings into ritual objects, elevating the Mantles, Namaths, and Aldrins beyond public scrutiny. Spectacle becomes imaginative balm for new wounds.

III

Sport is tied to industry because it represents a reaction to industry.[11] Baseball became the nation's favorite game during a violent, squalid industrialization. The game melded field with factory, incorporating the techniques of an emerging capitalism with a pastoral panorama. The sward of green turf still exists amidst the bleakness of the surrounding industrial tenements it was meant to deny. The pace, now too slow for an electronic age, promised long outdoor hours as an antidote to the boredom of industry:

> He jeers the officials and indulges in hot arguments with his neighbors, stamping and ranting. . . . All the time his vital organs are summoned into strenuous sympathy and he draws deep breaths of pure air. He may be weary when the game is over but for it he will eat and sleep better, his step will be more determined, his eyes will cease resembling those of a dead fish. . . . He goes back to his desk or bench next day with a smiling face.[12]

Baseball was not only an escape; it reinforced capitalist values. The game treated people as property. "Trading" and "bonuses" were means of improving efficiency and sharpening competition. Baseball also incorporated "stealing"—a risk proportional to an individual's ability and his luck. Industry increased production through standardization; so did baseball. Each player is a specialist;

the team (with its "manager" and "front office") became a protocorporation where the spectator could measure the output (of runs). Batting averages, earned-run averages were comforting percentages: simple calculations in a world of outrageous figures and complicated equations. Medieval pageants attested to the Church's accuracy; baseball affirmed the new world of accounting and double-entry bookkeeping. "It is good to care in any dimension," William Saroyan said about the national pastime. "More Americans put their spare (and purest?) caring into baseball." [13] Seymour Siwoff, the accountant who keeps the statistics for the National League, has a sign above his door: ETERNAL VIGILANCE IS THE PRICE OF ACCURACY IN STATISTICS. If baseball reduces people to numbers, the figures have, at least, a continuity and a relationship to the past. The faith in statistics prevents baseball from changing its rules because the hitting and pitching averages of the future would have no relationship to those of the past. The sentimental attachment to statistics is expressed by Siwoff in *Sports Illustrated* (August 18, 1969):

> What I enjoy most about statistics is the chance they give you to relive the past. When Ernie Banks gets seven RBIs in a game or when Reggie Jackson gets ten, it brings back memories of when Jim Bottomley drove in eleven. In looking up those things, I can see those guys as clearly as if they were playing again.

Invoking an uncomplicated past, statistics and the umpire's rule book bring the authority of "science" and "law" onto the field. The spectators and players respect both forces; they abide by a trained, "objective" decision. The game allows the illusion of freedom, but violent disagreement is not tolerated. Eccentricity, like Richie Allen's scribbling of words to the spectators in front of first base, is carefully patrolled. Allen is a renegade within a system that cannot tolerate friction. Baseball dramatizes acquiescence to system, law, and the mathematics of productivity.

IV

Technology creates its own demand. As America becomes increasingly systematized, unified, and efficient, the public wants more technique in its spectacles. Football offers a picture of the gorgeousness of enforced specialization of human effort. In the game, technique is concomitant with victory. Writing of coach Vince Lombardi, veteran guard Jerry Kramer stresses the importance of superhuman performance and accuracy:

> He makes us execute the same plays over and over, a hundred times, two hundred times, until we do every thing right automatically. He works to make the kickoff return team perfect. He ignores nothing. Technique, technique, technique, over and over and over, until we feel like we're going crazy. But we win.[14]

The football player's ability to make a machine of his body sustains the spectator's faith in technology. The drama of football pits man-and-technique against man-and-technique. Films, training devices, medical equipment, special diets reflect the game's reliance on scientific discovery for *protection, defense,* and *victory.* When a Miami Dolphin end received a second concussion, a special helmet was devised to protect him. Joe Namath's million-dollar knees are guarded by a specially constructed brace. Scientific innovation is part of the team's efficiency.

Football's appeal rests with the intricacy of its system. The game emphasizes a mechanized, industrial sense of time. The players "watch the clock"; seconds become dramatic divisions. Even the vocabulary of play is in mathematical language in which the offensive runner and his destination on the line of scrimmage are identified by number. Jerry Kramer mentions a "forty-nine sweep," which means that the number four back will take the ball into the "nine" hole, the area outside the right end.

Graceful, strong, fierce—the football player is an automaton in the world of action. Jerry Kramer describes the fatigue of training:

> All I know is that when everyone else moves, I move, and when everyone files on the bus, I get on the bus. . . . I really don't know what time it is, what day it is . . . I don't know anything at all.[15]

Joe Namath recounts the programing of new data ("automatics") on the line of scrimmage during the Super Bowl:

> When I change a play . . . they've got to drive the play they've been thinking about from their minds and they've got to replace it with a new one, and in a few seconds they've got to be ready for a different assignment, maybe on a different snap count, maybe in a whole different direction.[16]

The implications of football are hidden by the excitement. The game confirms America's abiding faith in technology as a means of progress. Football is a spectacle of superhuman effort attesting to the value of research, training, discipline, and refinement. There is a messianic atmosphere to football—the locker-room talks, the bravado of the spectators which brings them to their feet or sends them out into the field after a game to rip down the goal posts. Football is a triumph of technique and community. The spectacle offers an image of athletic unity and creates an emotional consensus:

> Technique provides a justification to everybody and gives all men the conviction that their actions are just, good, and in the spirit of truth. The individual finds the same conviction in his fellow workers and feels himself strengthened.[17]

V

Baseball and football make reality out of a game. The space race makes a game out of reality. Technology extends the demand, fed by sport, for continued, easy victory with no sacrifice from the community of observers. The Apollo 11 was described in terms of a game. The familiar features of sport facilitate public acquiescence to the awesome specter of the machine being willed to power over man. The astronauts are the gold-dust twins of the galaxies; their training is an athlete's regimen of diet, study, and drills. Neil Armstrong's statement in *Life* magazine (August 22, 1969) illustrates how the vocabulary becomes propaganda:

> This nation was depending on the NASA-industry team to do the job and that team was staking its reputation on Apollo 11. A lot of necks had been put voluntarily on the chopping block, and as more and more attention focused on the flight it became evident that any failure would bring certain tarnish to the U.S. image.

The moonshot is an instant image of progress in a society where social reform is thought to involve sacrifice: "Landing men on the moon has proven easier than unraveling problems such as public welfare." (*Life* magazine, August 22, 1969) Trained to witness gargantuan athletic feats, the American spectator accepts scientific hardware as matter-of-factly as a batting machine. The space program is its own justification:

> Modern men are so enthusiastic about technique, so assured of its superiority, so immersed in the technical milieu, that without exception they are oriented toward technical progress.[18]

The moonshot is the triumph of system. Aficionados of the moon spectacle can only applaud and succumb. Yet a new world has been spawned which will affect the way man works and how he relates to his environment. As a chauvinistic article in *Fortune* magazine (July 1969) testified:

> The really significant fallout from the strains, traumas, and endless experiment of Project Apollo has been . . . techniques for directing the massed endeavors of scores of thousands of minds in a close-knit mutually enhancive combination of government, university, and private industry.

The space game makes man wet nurse to machinery. Armstrong, Aldrin, and Collins manipulate dials. They were first on the moon, but there are dozens waiting in the wings who can do the same thing as efficiently. They do not fit the conventional heroic mold; their function is not total. They are not free, lone men grappling with a recalcitrant universe. Thousands of others are keeping them aloft. The hero is the machine, not man. As Michael Collins said, "The computer, of course, had been telling me that everything was going well. . . ." In the space game, as with all sports spectacles, man is the master of external details which have no bearing on his inner life. The technician's freedom is a slavery to machinery and the system that organizes it. Human value is compromised, the inner life devalued in the performance of tasks. Aldrin, discussing the content of his prayers during the moon trip, told *Life* magazine:

> I was not so selfish as to include my family in those prayers, nor so spacious as to include the fate of the world. I was thinking of our particular task and the challenge and opportunity that had been given us.

Aldrin, like the other astronauts, is programed to be a figure in a carefully constructed tableau. A prop instead of a person, his language is debased rather than destroyed by the technique that impels him to perform in the space spectacle.

The drama of teamwork, the tension of statistics and physical accuracy, are now firmly established in the real world as well as on the playing field. Spectacle overwhelms the senses. The astronauts are praised for characteristics which warp the human fiber. They represent in life the process that Americans cheer in the stadium:

> A new dismembering and a complete reconstruction of the human being so that he can at last become the objective (and also total object) of technique. He is also completely despoiled of everything that traditionally constitutes his essence. Man becomes pure appearance, a kaleidoscope of external shapes, an abstraction in a milieu that is frighteningly concrete . . . .

VI

Spectacle reinforces the illusion of objectivity. Events are paraded before the eye and the spectator feels imaginatively in control of both the game and its rules. Spectacle's clarity, its system, deny mystery:

> Technique worships nothing, respects nothing. It has a single role: to strip off externals, to bring everything to light, and by rational use to transform everything to means.

The nonrational, the defiant, the emotionally unpalatable must be dismissed and ultimately eliminated.

Theater cannot compete with the ritual experience of sports spectacle, but it can learn from it. As a handicraft industry in a technological age, theater has lost its sense of ritual and forgotten how to deal with primal impulses. Too often our theater is overly polite and self-conscious. It rarely understands the spectacle it offers and how to capitalize on the forms of pleasure which feed its audience's "collective unconscious." The fact of theater being a game is often forgotten in the attempt to make a serious statement. Yet the process of "gaming" can have a more profound effect on an audience than a narrative plot. Theater pieces like John Ford Noonan's *The Year Boston Won the Pennant*, Peter Terson's *Zigger Zagger* (soccer), David Storey's *The Changing Room* (rugby), and Arthur Kopit's *Indians* have a radical stage potential because they invoke memories of comfortable spectacle and mythic appeal, only to work against those assumptions. The spectator subsequently becomes aware that he is both dreamer and diminished man.

By understanding the force of spectacle, American theater can redefine itself more vigorously. It can be an island of humanity and freedom in a sea of banal uniformity and data. The axioms of a technological society cannot be answered by an equally pat denial; but the forms that make them acceptable to the public can be imaginatively exploded. Technology and the forces that promote it are too large to be reversed, but a countervailing theater may have a heroic destiny and a liberty the rest of America is losing.

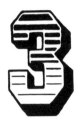

1789: The French Revolution
Year One

Avant-garde theater has always been inspired by a nostalgia for the memorable, makeshift wonders of the fairground. Alfred Jarry wanted Père Ubu to be a "man-sized marionnette." Meyerhold, in an essay significantly entitled "The Fairground Booth," touted the strolling player as the source "that keeps alive the true art of acting." Antonin Artaud, longing for a theater that would unleash radical energy through the danger and joy of irresistible movement and sound, found the epitome of his anarchist's dream in the Marx Brothers' improvised capers. All these innovators were actors looking for more flexible scenarios. The fairground represented a liberation from the conventions of production and performance: an adventure and a test. "The mime stops the mouth of the rhetorician who belongs not on the stage but in the pulpit; the juggler reveals the total self-sufficiency of the actor's skill with the expressiveness of his gesture and the language of his movements—not only in the dance but in his every step." [1]

1789, a spectacle of the first year of the French Revolution which I saw in a converted London warehouse and which was performed originally in a hangar on the outskirts of Paris, is an attempt to move theater forward by going back to the spirit and style of the fairground tradition. Created and performed with the high-amperage energy of good intentions by Le Théâtre du Soleil, *1789* does not turn history into a theater of intractable and numbing fact (80 per cent of the Third Estate illiterate; average life expectancy, twenty-nine years; factory working hours, 5 a.m.–7 p.m.). Instead, as reinterpreted by strolling players and performed for an audience which stands between five platforms stretched in a circle the size of a basketball court, it becomes a fairground show of skits, processions, and debates. As Irving Wardle, the critic for *The Times* of London observed:

> In structure and content it shows a series of waves of popular energy being checked by the successful returns to order. At first, the enemy is the artistocracy; at the end it is the bourgeoisie; but in every case the people are cheated into renewed servitude by yet another repressive regime. The phrase *la Révolution est finie* resounds through the show like a death knell.[2]

What is exciting about *1789* is its attempt to find new theatrical forms to assess history. Documentary facts are never enough to touch the soul of an audience. On stage, the arithmetics of atrocity neither instruct nor delight. The certainty of numbers leaves the stage static, and our minds strangely unprovoked. Le Théâtre du Soleil wants to get into our dreams. The fairground is a resonant setting for this. "We knew it would be a fairground: a form which is simple and popular, which existed at that time, and before

and after that time," [3] explains the director Ariane
Mnouchkine. The fairground, in other words, brings with it
a history of its own. The shared memory of its tradition is
part of the method through which political theater can
launch its attack on the historical assumptions of the society. Radical theater has always wanted to make a seismic
disturbance in its audience. But this cannot be done by but-
tonholing an audience or bludgeoning it; or, sadly, by performing for ten people on a street corner. To touch and
transform the popular imagination, the theater must em-
ploy forms which can have a wide popular appeal. The
story of the Revolution is, to the Frenchman, as vivid and
familiar as Paul Revere's ride.

The fairground's appeal is also in the democracy of its
audience: people coming together and learning from
watching each other's reactions to events. Miss Mnouchkine
says:

> Of the public that does come, I doubt whether there is har-
> mony between the 1,000 people in the house. We get di-
> vided reactions. Protest generally takes the form of silence
> because the majority is young and enthusiastic. We've had
> *Vive le Roi* a few times. Nobody yet has shouted *Vive la bour-
> geoisie,* which would be a pretty poor slogan. When we have
> played to working-class spectators we find they've been very
> respectful and attentive. And then they ask questions of
> fact: Is that true, is that dangerous, how is that made? [4]

I

Like all street theater, *1789* makes a grotesque of history.
The grotesque is a means of participating in tragedy but,
through irony, escaping its emotional consequence. Low

comedy mingles with social outrage. With several actors playing the King and Queen—with historical figures caricatured—*1789* declares its focus to be the patterns of history rather than the motives of individual characters. Kenneth Tynan, in a debate following a performance in London, argued:

> Our theatre suffers from the fact that it is mostly concerned with the intimate private problems of middle-class people, and that is exactly the sort of theatre and film which has been crippling an attempt to expand and extend the nature of human responses in an auditorium. What Ariane's approach does is to explode out from the individual centrifugally; and it seems to me that an individual writing a play about history tends to see it always in terms of individual psychology. . . . He puts himself into the mind of a character, and of course sympathizes with the character more than with others, and so the whole movement of history becomes seen in terms of three or four individuals. What a collective approach does is [to never allow us] to concentrate on [an] individual['s] problems, his pathos, his tragedies, but on the problems of whole classes, whole social groups. And it is precisely by getting outside the individual psyche, by abandoning individual focus, that the broad movement of history becomes possible in the theatre, perhaps for the first time.[5]

Tynan responds to the intention of the production, but not the result.

The style of *1789* matches the political excesses of the time—as exaggerated in performance as the common man's poverty and the nobility's lavishness. The audience is not plunged into revolution; but led, carefully, through it. *1789* creates a theatrical revolution as rational and mechanistic as Descartes' God. Events rarely swirl around us; they progress logically from platform to platform. The complex plot-

points of the Revolution force the production to languish in
tableaux vivants that illustrate rather than dramatize, and
leave history, in its simplification, not clarified but confused. The play's final upbeat words are given to Gracchus
Babeuf, the radical leader, haranguing for the Revolution:

> . . . May the people turn all the ancient and barbarous in-
> stitutions upside down! May the hideous war of the rich
> against the poor cease to be such that all the audacity is on
> one side and all the cowardice is on the other. Yes, I say
> again, the tide of evil is full; things cannot get any worse.
> They cannot be put right except by total overthrow.
>
> Let's see the end of society as it is! Let's see the happiness
> of the common people. After a thousand years, let's come at
> last to change these rank, stupid laws.

But Babeuf, the man Alexander Herzen dubbed a "mas-
todon of socialism," would six years later propose strict authoritarian control of the populace. The concept of a people's freedom was rhetoric: equality was a revolutionary
illusion. As Herzen writes, "Decrees of the government provided for, have survived, with their heading: Égalité, Li-
berté, Bonheur Commun, to which was added, by way of
elucidation, 'Ou la mort!' " [6]

A polemic theater must be unfair. Its first premise is that
our ways of understanding the past and what is accepted
from the past are faulty. So, to default *1789*, as John
Weightman did, on the ground of historical inaccuracy is to
miss the point of the spectacle:

> Why give such importance to Cagliostro, who was a minor
> symptom? Why, if post-1789 events are included, not give
> the September Massacres, the Feast of Reason, the execu-
> tion of André Chénier, and a dozen other attractively theat-
> rical episodes. Anyone who actually knows something about

the Revolution can only be puzzled; anyone who doesn't will have his head stuffed with misconceptions.[7]

Excellence lies in staying within the spirit of the facts. As with any street theater, it is not the poetry or the power of words which dazzle the imagination and linger in the memory, but the evocative clarity and sharpness of the stage images. Street theater trades in essences. To be persuasive, its images must be irrefutable. To penetrate the public imagination, these images must be as vivid as dreams. Miss Mnouchkine shocked English critics—as wedded to a literary theater as Chevalier to his boater—when she admitted in debate, "We made the play as simple as we could. We think it is not simple enough." [8] When *1789* fails, it is because the production does not compress and refine emotions. A storyteller begins the evening with five exemplary fables of oppression. Each tale blurs with the next; the effect is to numb the audience rather than surprise it:

> Listen, if you will, to the story of Mary, called Mary the Miserable, who was born old and miserable like her mother and grandmother before her, in a country inhabited by two ogres. . . .
>
>> *(Music of Johann Sebastian Bach)*
>> THE PRELATE: May God bless this house!
>> THE LORD: And may my arms protect it.
>> THE PRELATE: My tithe!
>> THE LORD: My dues.
>> *(They tear her pot away from her. She screams her revolt and her misery, her hands outstretched toward the audience public which she thus engages as witness. Her cry fades, the light dims, the* STORYTELLER *continues. . . .)*

The audience is momentarily given the role of witness;

but as a group it cares most when scenes—in their bravado
—capture more fully the emotional truth of a moment. At
one point, we watch the Third Estate being swindled by
politicians in a hilarious puppet show—the Common Man
is batted down by the Nobility and the Clergy with Punch
and Judy's coy but consistent violence. We listen, at another moment in this prismatic presentation, to three peasants as they joyfully respond to the news that they can write
the King a list of their grievances.

NESTINE: I begin with the Salt-Tax!

MARY: Oh, yes! Salt-Tax to the King.

NESTINE: I need a pen. *(They run after an imaginary hen and
    pluck a feather)* I write "Salt-Tax" what will I use for ink?

GASPARD: Something black.

NESTINE: I've got no black.

ALL *(to the public)*: Haven't you got anything black, white,
    or red.

NESTINE: Gaspard! Something red. We need blood then!

GASPARD: That's it. Cut me!

NESTINE: I shall not cut you for the Salt-Tax.

MARY: Go on. *(Gaspard cuts himself, Nestine hugs him, dips her
    pen in the blood and prepares to write)*

NESTINE: I am writing "Salt-Tax" to the King. *(Hesitates)*
    How do you make an "S"?

GASPARD: Write "Salt-Tax."

NESTINE: Okay. You write it. I don't even know how to
    make an "S."

ALL: How do you make an "S"? If you haven't written any-
    thing down, we won't be able to change anything.

This kind of sketch, with its possibility for comic charac-
terization as well as irony, has a satiric edge. It is people's
theater that speaks to the ordinary man with both the

humor which helps him survive and the anger which, besides his body, he knows is his only resource.

The actors make a few sallies into the audience. Mammoth puppet representations of the King and Queen—their robes floating dramatically behind them—run through the auditorium. The actors parade as the new *petite bourgeoisie*, debating the idea of social order as they move from one platform to another. But there is very little authentic emotional contact with the spectators. Occasionally, as when the actors splinter among the audience telling the same story of the events leading up to the storming of the Bastille, *1789* creates the sense of intimacy and passion of strolling players. Here the audience takes on a genuine character in the spectacle. We strain close, as the peasants must have done, to hear the latest news.

. . . A boy even put nails in his gun, that shows you the state we were in. Then an idea struck us: all the guns, powder, and bullets we wanted were at—guess where?—the Bastille. And the Bastille represented what we didn't want. It represented authority, despotism, its guns were aimed at the Faubourg Saint-Antoine, where we lived. . . . So we went to the Bastille and its governor, DeLaunay, and told him: "Give us arms, DeLaunay." He didn't want to give us any and he put the Bastille in a state of defense. . . . Ah well, we attacked it, we people of Paris: there was a boy, a wheelwright, who crossed over the kitchen roof and let down the drawbridge. Then we were engulfed in the first courtyard—pow! pow! pow!—they fired on us from above. Our hearts were uplifted. A delegation from the Hôtel de Ville came with a white hat to parlay. We let them through. Then the soldiers fired on them from above, a delegation with a white hat! Then we said, so it's like that, so much the worse, there will be more dead and wounded, they will fill up the ditches and we will be able to pass. It will make us more fiery. And we came to the second courtyard. There was more smoke. We couldn't see anything any more. We would still have been in that position if the Invalides had not taken pity on us. They refused to continue firing on us, laid down their arms, and forced DeLaunay to capitulate. And that's how we, the people of Paris, took the Bastille.

The rhythm of this speech mounts—voices shriek, kettle-drums roll. A man rushes to a platform. "Citizens," he declares. "THE PEOPLE HAVE WON." The moment is gorgeous; the tension bursts into full-scale celebration with juggling, dancing, wrestling. The jarring shift from the claustrophobic intimacy of the peasants' narrative to carnival is the most original and disconcerting moment in the spectacle. It is exciting because in a gesture we witness the kind of flexibility environmental theater can achieve: making use of the entire auditorium not just the stage, of the people not just the players. But having once lured the audience into the role of common man—asking us to step up and try the wheel of fortune, throwing hats on broomsticks, and winning rosettes for our marksmanship—the spectacle pulls back from any real theatrical risk. At a moment when there should be dancing in the streets, we have only an actor in a bear costume, dancing with an actress. Unlike *Orlando Furioso*, the prototype of these popular environmental events and a healthy and strong influence on this production, *1789* has no real intention of sustaining the audience's role in the play; or, of sustaining a fairground sense of wonder. Miss Mnouchkine explains:

> I don't like this expression, "use the audience." It was a big discovery on the first night to see how beautiful the public was. But we didn't intend to use them. We use ourselves for

them. Our first intention was to be freer; which doesn't happen of course because there are usually too many people.
But at the first few performances in Milan, when we had
only about 600, it was incredible to see how the audience
did move around, to get in closer and make its own picture.[9]

But the nature of the production—its mobility, its special
drama, its narrative—demands a continual involvement
and manipulation of the audience. The failure of the production to feel this need is a major lapse of directorial judgment.

Spatially, what promises to be an exciting environmental
experiment finally fizzles out. Although the spirit of the
production and the environment seem to want a revolution
in a way of performing and producing plays, most of the
events could as easily be performed on a proscenium stage.
We stand to watch the spectacle and need only turn our
heads to see what happens next. Instead of learning the
rules of the play by grappling with the uniqueness of the
production, exploring it the way children do a playground,
a preshow announcement asks us to kindly refrain from sitting on the stages or the connecting footbridges. This the
audience should discover by playing with the company. If
spectators get in the way, they should be pushed off. *1789*
has style but no danger, energy but no obsession. Miss
Mnouchkine's direction is incredibly ambitious, but it
promises more than it produces. The event takes on a formal control and logical progression which are at odds with
the spectacle's desire to astound. Collectively created, *1789*
is weighted down by too many vignettes that indulge the actors' discoveries but add little to our sense of the Revolution.
Miss Mnouchkine wants content, but in her enthusiastic innocence does not understand that form itself carries a very

strong meaning. "Our aim is to tell as clearly as possible a story which all French people know already. . . . The pleasure and magic of *Orlando Furioso* is in space organization, not content." [10] Archetypes of literature (*Orlando*) or history (*1789*) are shared by a public imagination: to use and to inform them demands the economy and cunning which Miss Mnouchkine and her troupe are on the way to developing.

II

Le Théâtre du Soleil, even with its failures, is more satisfying and more provocative than most conventional theater. Its appeal indicates the shifting attitudes toward theatrical production. Conventional plays rarely challenge the intellect or the performer's acting mechanism. The economics of production also enforce a kind of censorship. Le Théâtre du Soleil exists outside the conventional patterns of stage art and economics. The group is fighting an artistic battle first outlined by Meyerhold in 1910. "Symbolic figures, processions, battles, prologues, parades: they are all elements of that pure theatricality which even the mysteries could not do without." [11] The time is right for the revolution Meyerhold defined a half-century ago. The fairground acrobat is more versatile than the matinee idol; the noise and excitement of a milling crowd more stimulating than a polite intermission. If Le Théâtre du Soleil's actors need training and experience, they are, at least, directing their energies more creatively, finding a future in reviving the performing tradition of the past. Meyerhold's indictment of theater is implicit in the aspirations of *1789*:

> In the contemporary theatre the comedian has been replaced by the "educated reader." "The play will be read in

costume and make-up" might as well be the announcement on playbills today. The new actor manages without the mask and the technique of the juggler. The mask has been replaced by make-up which facilitates representation of every feature of the face as it is observed in real life. The actor has no need of the juggler's art, because he no longer "plays" but simply "lives" on the stage. "Play-acting," that magic word of theater, means nothing to him because as an imitator he is incapable of rising to the level of improvisation which depend on infinite combinations and variations of all the tricks at the actor's command.[12]

1789 points the way toward a theater of authentic, fulfilling play. Le Théâtre du Soleil, if it can stay together, is capable of creating great work. Already, *1789* has been dubbed by the London *Times* "a work of international importance." In terms of intention, yes; but accomplishment, no. The ingredients for a radical theater are here: courage, intelligence, tenacity, and a sense of fun. The fairground performance is on its way back: its glitter and noise a healthy antidote to the swamp of words and tepid gestures which pass for "drama" in the conventional playwright's theater. Where American theater is corrupted and killed by shaky economic foundations, Mnouchkine's theater is attempting to make a clean break with the commercial structure. "What happens before a play reaches the public has nothing to do with me," protested one listener at Miss Mnouchkine's discussion. Her reply is typical of the exemplary effort of Le Théâtre du Soleil:

It is as much your concern to know how this play has been done as it is to know that the sugar you drink in your coffee or your tea has been acquired out of the slavery of somebody. It is exactly the same concern. To know that a certain product can be made without any sensation of oppression, or slavery, or exploitation is an important fact which must concern you.[13]

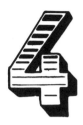

Andre Gregory's
Alice in Wonderland:
Playing with Alice

In the sphere of sacred play, the child and the
poet are at home with the savage.
　　—J. HUIZINGA, *Homo Ludens*

Alice in Wonderland is a playful, elusive fable. For psychologists, her world is a textbook on schizophrenia, a study in repression; for literary sleuths, religious and historical allegories loom out of every weird encounter like the Cheshire Cat's grin. Perhaps the profoundest interpretation is the simplest: the tale is a game. Carroll conceived his stories in a convivial mood, entertaining his beloved Alice Liddell and her sisters in their rides up the Cherwell. The scenes are preoccupied with riddles, debates, contests, and reveal not only his passion for young ladies, but his understanding of the nature of play. *Alice* is not simply an innocent, optimistic yarn; her condition in Wonderland is more ominous. Yet the literary delights and memorable situations in the tale have become so familiar that the quality of Alice's experience is often overlooked. This is a play world; but a game "incorporates an *agon*—hence our agony—a struggle." [1] In Wonderland, Alice has the symptoms of a modern urban malaise. She is homeless, forgetful, nostalgic, fragmented, emotionally and physically warped. She enters the unknown—a world with special rules that are neither safe nor predictable. Each confrontation is a contest demanding risk and stamina.

Play demands discipline, concentration, endurance, and skill. When a child plays, he is testing the world. He also enters a world apart from his normal one. The appeal of play is its quality of intuitive discovery, its existence outside the domination of any system but its own. Play is an activity beyond self-consciousness and conventional judgment. Tension is crucial to play. "Who will win?" "What will happen?" "Can he do it?" This anxiety turns action into enchantment, accomplishment into wonder. As Johan Huizinga writes, "The more difficult the game, the greater the tension in the beholders." [2]

Alice in Wonderland is constructed on one fundamental tension: the spirit of play. Its conventional image evolves from the famous John Tenniel illustrations that accompany Carroll's text. The sketches have a sedate, adult's view of the fantasy—neat, witty, whimsical but not outrageous, vigorous but not violent. The Victorian precision of Tenniel's drawings have influenced both film and earlier stage versions which aspired to imitate the detail and action, but not the central source of energy. We are accustomed to Alice in her pinafore, the Mad Hatter dressed like an Old

Etonian. But the magic of Carroll's fantasy draws its zest from the child's ability in play to transform himself, to conjure objects, to play with an earnestness which accepts the visionary world.

Andre Gregory's version of *Alice in Wonderland* (which incorporates scenes from *Through the Looking Glass*) returns the fable to its vulnerable confrontations and playfulness. By imposing a physical theatrical style on Carroll's text, Gregory unlocks *Alice*'s mystery. The fable becomes a new game, not a set piece. Gregory's production is the most thorough and intelligent application of performance theory to a classical text yet evolved in America. The power and importance of Gregory's *Alice* lies not only in its fresh evocation of the tale, but in its disciplined modification of the acting techniques of Jerzy Grotowski. Much American avant-garde theater has borne his imprint. Typical of our consumer society, Grotowski's ideas have been devoured but not digested. Gregory uses Grotowski as a foundation for theatrical discovery:

> Many people try to imitate Grotowski. They learn the wrong lessons. For me, the lesson of Grotowski is his emphasis on the details in a production. Every single detail is specific and clear like in a painting or sculpture. Finished, chiseled, selected, and perfect. Spiritually, I think he's of great importance because he emphasizes that you must always go further—physically, mentally, socially. You must always destroy what you've done before. Each time you must destroy yourself in order to live again. Some of his exercises are of value; but even he drops them. His exercises grow out of specific productions.
>
> —GREGORY, in a conversation

Grotowski has pointed a way toward freeing the theater

from the mundane and inauthentic. He has written: "The theater must recognize its own limitations. If it cannot be richer than the cinema, then let it be poor. If it cannot be as lavish as television, let it be ascetic. If it cannot be a technical attraction, let it renounce all outward technique." [3] Grotowski's work exhibits the modern (and very American) yearning to conjure, through performance, a new psychic unity, a union of mind with body, of action with mystery. The philosophy behind his performance theory meshes startlingly with Alice's condition in Wonderland. Gregory has control of Grotowski's techniques and has matched them with a text which also has its root in excessive "play." The style is itself a point of view. The stage is swept clean of all but the most utilitarian props. The emphasis is on confrontation. Alice's struggles to establish her identity and to connect with the topsy-turvy creatures she encounters parallel the need behind performance theater. Both test and show the resourcefulness, the courage, the freedom, and imaginative possibilities of the human will.

Alice confronts characters who have no apparent motivation. Their personalities surprise Alice; their uniqueness, their rigorous demands are a challenge to her. The audience, like Alice, discovers them in the purity of their outrageous presence. Grotowski's teaching emphasizes this playful immediacy. Performance theater breaks down the masks which make-up, elaborate costume, and conventional gesture impose on the theatrical event. The actor is exposed, not hidden behind props. Grotowski's minimal impulse emphasizes the existential fact of the actor: he is there. Theater comes back to game—the spectacle, the competition, the physical drama of the actor versus the demands of the text. His prowess must inspire awe; his visible presence must elevate a fiction into an actuality. "To be present is to be ready to dispose of oneself, to give oneself, to make a present of oneself, to fill the emptiness that aches." [4] Grotowski's *exercice plastique* systematizes the creation of this sense of visible presence.

Wonderland is surreal; events and people, in Alice's words, become "curiouser and curiouser." The people Alice discovers are in an obsessive, spiritual state. The Caterpillar is stoned. The Hatter and March Hare are crazy. The White Knight is possessed by his own inventions. The White Queen is *distraite,* frantic about tomorrow, and unable to conceive of today; she is totally lost in time. The unnaturalness of the environment, and the unusual psychic conditions of the characters also mesh with crucial ingredients of Grotowski's theory. Grotowski argues that there should be nothing "natural" (representational) in acting. "At a moment of psychic shock, a moment of terror, of mortal danger or tremendous joy, a man does not behave naturally. A man in an elevated spiritual state uses articulated signs, begins to dance, to sing. . . ." [5] Gregory applies this impulse to the text, and endows it with a new kind of performance freedom. He succeeds in creating a sense of presence and, with it, the danger and the surprise of bearing witness to the human spirit fulfilling its dream of possibility.

> We have physical blocks. There are areas of our body that we don't express with but we don't know why. Take the most obvious example—a girl who is shy about expressing with her bosom. Somebody trained in method acting like Lee Strasberg would say: "Darling, the reason you're inhibited is because as a child . . ." Grotowski says screw that. Commit your breasts, and in committing them you find the nerve to express through that part of the body. His exercises

are marvelous for training the actor not to be physical but to express with every part of his body. It is a new kind of freedom. Who's interested in just being physical? What I wanted to do was create actors, who because they could express with their whole body, exist on a kind of dream level. But in ordinary life, we express only with our eyes, our voice, and our hands. Everything between is cut off most of the time. . . .

—GREGORY, in a conversation

In this physical challenge, the actor (not just the text) enters the unknown. Actions become dangerous and risky. In Wonderland, nothing holds its shape. Alice is transformed, and so is the world around her. She becomes small, then large, then small again. Figures loom out at her from strange angles and take on menacing proportions. The fable's mystery is equaled by the magic of a physical performance in which a gesture has its own beauty and meaning, only to vanish with the next image. "Impulse and action are concurrent: The body vanishes, burns, and the spectator sees only visible impulses." [6] Grotowski's words could describe the kaleidoscopic quality of Wonderland. The gestures of Gregory's production occur with such rapid clarity that, like play, what is remembered is the sense of energy. The mystery is preserved; the unusual actions play against the familiarity of the text. "How will they do the Caterpillar?" "How is Alice going to get through a small door when there is no set?" This sense of anticipation feeds the tension, the wonder, and the excitement. Like the riddles and word games in *Alice*, the stage event becomes a puzzle which the audience must "solve."

Wonderland is also a very special place. Any serious "playing" must have its unique area. Grotowski has a brilliant intuition of this essential dynamic of play, maximizing the tension between audience and event by carefully modulating the space surrounding them. In his *Dr. Faustus*, the audience sat at banquet tables on which the play took place. In *The Constant Prince*, the audience was above the action, peering down like interns in an operating theater at the Prince's sacrifice. For a performing theory which aspires to rejuvenate our concept of play, there must be a well chosen, unique *playground:* "a forbidden spot, isolated, hedged round, hallowed, within which special rules obtain." [7]

II

To enter Gregory's Wonderland, the audience, like Alice, must symbolically burrow into a new world. The audience crowds into an outer room filled with cookies and lemonade under the caveats DRINK ME, EAT ME. These words, which transform Alice in size, begin the audience's reinitiation into the realm of child's play. The room is connected to the play area by a small door. The spectators bend through it, entering the space one at a time. Inside, a parachute umbrellas out like a circus tent, buttressed by wooden beams and white rope. Half big top and half tree house, the space is claustrophobic. The audience sits on bleacher seats and on the floor. "I wanted to create for the audience what I had gone through creating the play—a return to childhood, a feeling in the audience that they were going back." But Gregory's environment for Wonderland is neither lip-smacking nor golden. There is no pastoral clutter. Wonderland is barren, tacky, and threatening. An antique gramophone, its trumpet blossoming out ominously like a tropical plant, is hinged to a tent pole. Carroll's Victorian bower is transformed into a no man's land. The back wall is a curtain of newspapers. When the actors enter, they burst through the paper like circus clowns. The characters emerge literally out of print to be reconstructed through performance before our eyes. The actors are not realistic replicas of Carroll's fable. Their costumes acknowledge a relationship to the text, and to the physical training performance theater requires.

> I wanted to give a sense that these were the things they played in, the clothes they worked in: A kind of bizarre work clothes. The textures are all things like quilts and mattress padding, which have associations with beds and lunatic asylums. It's almost as if you had a group of kids who had walked into a padded cell and taken the padding off the walls and made costumes.
>
> —GREGORY, in a conversation

The costumes, the new gestures, the rearrangement of the text disorient the audience. The group of performers surrounds Alice, crushing her inside them, holding a jagged umbrella like a bird's wing. They chant the nonsense words of "Jabberwocky." Alice fends off the violent, suffocating yet seductive words that smother her: "Frumious bandersnatch," "the vorpal blade went snicker-snack." She enters a terrain where fun implies madness, where to play is to risk one's self. Gregory forces Alice to emerge not simply from good-natured frolic, but from private pain and humming confusion.

Alice is terrorized, victimized, befriended. On Alice's journey, games are the only means of surviving; her only hope is through playing with the creatures in Wonderland. The game world is an adjustment to new, authoritarian rules. "Play demands order absolute and supreme." [8] Each pressure on Alice nurtures the atmosphere of violence. Gregory's images spiral and compound as Alice games her way through Wonderland. Her final encounter with the White Knight is the meanest and most upsetting. In Carroll's tale, the Knight is passive; here, the Knight uses every tactic to keep Alice playing. Alice "doesn't want to play." The Knight forces her. "Guard against the bite of sharks." He nips at Alice's leg. "I hope you've got your hair well fastened on?" He pulls her hair. The Knight tries to stuff Alice into an imaginary bag, to eliminate the "kill-joy."

The ultimate game impulse is the play's physical transformations in the performances. The hole down which Alice disappears is conjured by bodies stacked one on top of another to receive her. Carroll's bizarre landscape is given its physical correlative. In the text, Alice simply tumbles down the hole. In Gregory's production, her tortuous descent is shown. The audience sees her whirled about, floating through the air, toppling into her underworld. When she surfaces at the end of the play, these actions are repeated— but backward. In these minimal surroundings, the spectator's imagination invents an entire physical world for Alice. The garden door, to which she lacks the key and is too large to enter, is created by an actor with his thumb and forefinger. The backs of actors form the mushroom on which the Caterpillar sits. The hookah that the Caterpillar smokes with stoned aplomb is the arm of an actor playing the mushroom. The Caterpillar puffs at his thumb. No shape stays the same. Bodies become croquet balls, wickets, forests, animals, balloons. One game merges with another. Alice is not only involved in finding a way out of the labyrinth, but in competing in local sports: a Caucus Race, a

Tea Party which ends in a spitting match, a game of toss with an egg on a blanket which leads her to Humpty Dumpty. By being so true to the pure, violent earnestness of play, Gregory's production becomes disturbing, setting off ideas which plumb an audience's historical consciousness, its "historical ego." (Grotowski)

III

"It was much pleasanter at home," thought poor Alice, "when one wasn't always growing larger and smaller and being ordered about by mice and rabbits."

Like Alice, the society's sense of its imaginative size changes, but by current events, not magic. When dissent can affect government policy, American youth can feel themselves giants. Jerry Rubin, in remembering 1965 ("Then we were conquerors of the world"), indulges a heroic fantasy in writing an appeal for financial support before the conspiracy trial:

> The Romans slaughtered all the slaves, but the moral example lives on. . . . When the Roman Army came to kill Spartacus they faced a mass of thousands of slaves. They demanded Spartacus step forward.
>   "I am Spartacus!" shouted one slave.
>   "No, I am Spartacus!" shouted another.
>   "No, I am Spartacus!"
>   "No, I am Spartacus!"
>
> —*New York Review of Books*

Rubin imagines a spiritual unity. But when protest is disparaged and contained, when identity is denied in the same way Alice is frustrated by Tweedledum and Tweedledee or the Caterpillar, people are reduced imaginatively to the stature of impotent dwarfs. The psychic shock breeds paranoia. Among radicals who, like Alice, have found themselves "underground," there is much talk of being "invisible" but also surfacing with godlike power. A "Weather Report" from Bernardine Dohrn epitomizes the obsession. Announcing a Weatherman bombing in a fortnight, she taunts her readers with her sense of a Weatherman's ubiquity. "The rest of us move freely in and out of every youth scene in this country. We're not hiding; but we're invisible." [9] Like Alice, she is passing through repressive terrain. Alice's words echo with a modern complaint, "I can't stand it any longer . . . I can't explain myself because I'm not myself." Alice yanks the food off the Queen's table; Dohrn would blast it to smithereens. The frustration, the struggle for identity in a lunatic world which logically refuses to acknowledge it, are the same. Both want to understand and survive their particular societies' games. Both are playful. Child's play—its tests, challenges, firm rules—becomes an illuminating motif for most of contemporary life. The games in Gregory's production lead an audience to understand the dynamic of a "civilized" society. Justice is based on a competitive "adversary system"; war is fought according to rules set down by the Geneva Convention. Play becomes the basis for the structure of law, government, discourse, poetry, battle. Even President Nixon's justification for entering Cambodia is inspired by the idea of play. His rationale is couched in terms of "rules" and "challenge":

> Does the richest and strongest nation in the history of the world have the character to meet a direct challenge by a

group which rejects every effort to win a just peace, ignores our warning, tramples on solemn agreements. . . .

—*The New York Times*

Alice is continually pitted against figures of outrageous authority. "Who are you?" asks the Caterpillar. Alice isn't sure. Later, Tweedledum makes it clear that Alice has no identity and no direction. "If [Tweedledee] left off dreaming about you, where do you suppose you'd be. . . . You'd be nowhere. Why, you're only a sort of thing in his dream. . . ." Alice finally resorts to screaming, "I am real." This fear of not being seen and experienced is a frightening reality in America. When President Nixon can call student dissidents "bums," and Daniel Moynihan suggests "benign neglect" of ghetto areas, government is tacitly denying the pain, commitment, and helplessness of millions of Americans. Protest is a way of saying, "I am real." But often, the experience of American youth is as much a sense of dream as Alice's. When Abbie Hoffman approached the bench to make his final statement at the Chicago conspiracy trial, he spoke for a generation. During the trial, the prosecution, trying to prove their fatuous charge of conspiracy, asked him what he was wondering when he stood outside a building.

And I said, "Wonder? Wonder? I have never been on trial for wondering. Is that like a dream?" The prosecution said, "Yes, that's like a dream." And I have never been on trial for my dreams before. How can I respect the highest court in the land or a federal government that puts people on trial for their dreams? . . .[10]

Not only was Hoffman on trial for his dreams, he—like all the conspirators—found himself a victim of society's dream about him. The frustration and confusion can be read not only in the victims' faces but in a society where the number of domestic bombings—over 2500 during the Nixon Administration—is a barometer of the impotence and anger official indifference breeds. Alice's anger and confusion at the Mad Tea Party comes when she sees a space at a table though the March Hare and the Hatter insist there is no room. This situation is a paradigm of the madness of our society in which the poor see a Land of Plenty, as well as the injustice of privilege. When Alice is offered wine, she is suspicious:

> "I don't see any wine. . . ."
> "There isn't any," said the March Hare.
> "Then it wasn't very civil of you to offer it. . . ."

A similar mad, frustrating game is played out by American society which holds it to be self-evident that "life, liberty, and the pursuit of happiness" are everyone's due, while denying justice and civil rights.

Behind every flamboyant game in Gregory's production is a sense of betrayal. Alice is faced not only with the irresponsibility of authority, but the gibberish which passes for advice. This linguistic stalemate is one of the finest accomplishments of Gregory's production. Bodies and events become a macabre, outlandish vision, and the cornerstones of reason—logic and the word—are turned on their heads.

> "I don't want to go among mad people," Alice remarked.
> "Oh, you can't help that," said the Cat; "we're all mad here. I'm mad. You're mad."

The Cheshire Cat's statement is funny and strangely true. Everyone is warped by the abrasions of society. The Hatter and the March Hare have a civilized discussion, but the logical connectives are missing. Alice's astonishment and apprehension are similar to those of the young protesters visited by President Nixon in the early morning hours before the Washington March on May 10, 1970:

> No, he wasn't making any argument. That was the point. . . . He wasn't making any sense; he was just rambling about things that didn't make any sense, that didn't relate. . . . It was a surreal scene. . . . And people were asking him questions, and it was like he didn't hear them at all. He ignored them. . . . He was really in a fog. . . . He kept saying to us, have a nice day here, enjoy yourself . . . I'll tell the people not to bother you. Say what you want and really enjoy yourself and really it seemed as if he thought we were on a picnic.[11]

In Carroll's fiction, and in contemporary American life, language is reduced to nonsense, cut off from experience and from logic, yet furiously sincere. Andre Gregory's *Alice* becomes a resilient metaphor for the deep, inarticulate wounds our country endures. Inundated with official justifications, promises, explanations in the face of undeniable injustice and failure, language is divested of its credibility. President Nixon sends troops into Cambodia claiming the action was *not* an "invasion." The whole vernacular of existence becomes distorted. Peace means war; law and order means repression. Freedom means conformity. Protection of life means destruction of life. Every declared victory turns out to be a moral defeat. Alice's confrontation with Humpty Dumpty outlines this process of delusion from Judge Hoffman's court to Richard Nixon's politics.

> "When I use a word," Humpty Dumpty said in a rather scornful tone, "it means just what I choose it to mean—neither more nor less."

"The question is," said Alice, "whether you can make words mean so many different things?"

"The question is," said Humpty Dumpty, "which is to be master—that's all. . . ."

Language—the basis of communication—becomes a game. Alice's dilemma—her lost direction, her homelessness—parallels that of Samuel Beckett's hobos in *Waiting for Godot*. In Wonderland, Alice is faced with brain teasers, nonsense songs, parodies, conundrums. Similarly, with Vladimir and Estragon, the verbal games create a brittle but authentic community between the players. Vladimir and Estragon play their linguistic games to pass the time: burlesques, parodies, boastings, debates. These "canters" gloss their fear: their sense of the void outside the momentary excitement of their verbal sport. Language helps survive the loneliness, a dark impulse which is shared by Carroll's Alice:

Dear, dear! How queer everything is today! And yesterday things went on just as usual. I wonder if I've been changed in the night.

Vladimir is no more certain of his world than Alice.

Was I sleeping while the others suffered? Am I sleeping now? Tomorrow, when I wake, or think I do, what shall I say of today?

IV

Andre Gregory's *Alice in Wonderland* succeeds in evoking a dream consciousness. Like a Bosch painting, man and animal coexist with a brilliant, outrageous detail. Objects are catapulted into our field of vision with an unpredictable complexity, mixing the horrible with the hilarious. At a moment of imaginative torture (the Mad Tea Party), the Dormouse slumps drowsily, stuffing his mouth with bread, cringing from the Hatter's wallops with an Italian loaf when he tries to speak. The low comic melds with the high seriousness of the performers' discipline and the intensity of the playing. Gregory's production took two years to rehearse (and cost only two thousand dollars). The beauty of this labor is always visible. His actors—students from New York University—bring a flexibility and intelligence to their performance. Inventing a playfulness which clarifies our world without explaining it, the stage event goes beyond rationality. This is a pageant of movement, language, and invention; a ritual of games which brings both actor and audience back to the roots of their imaginative beginnings, their source of despair and joy. In choosing *Alice*, Gregory has incarnated Grotowski's intentions for Americans perhaps better than his mentor. For the meaning and appeal of his stage *Alice* lies finally in the mythic consciousness; the playful, primitive level we all share "where the child, the animal, the savage, and the seer belong in the region of dream, enchantment, ecstasy, and laughter." [12]

PLAYWRIGHTS

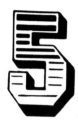

Pinter and Chekhov:
The Bond of Naturalism

We begin with the idea that nature is all we
need; it is necessary to accept her as she is,
without modifying her or diminishing her in
any respect; she is sufficiently beautiful and
great to provide a beginning, a middle, and
an end. Instead of imagining an adventure,
complicating it, and arranging a series of
theatrical effects to lead to a final conclusion,
we simply take from life the story of a being
or a group of beings whose acts we faithfully
set down. The work becomes an official
record, nothing more; its only merit is that of
exact observation, of the more or less
profound penetration of analysis, of the
logical concatenation of facts. . . .

—ÉMILE ZOLA, "On Naturalism
in the Theatre" (1880)

Naturalism has its roots in a scientific approach which melds man inextricably to his environment, studying him as a complex amalgam of audible rhythms and spectacular mutations for survival. Chekhov, himself a doctor, applied this discipline to the ailing conventional drama of his time.

> The demand is made that the hero and heroine should be dramatically effective. But in life people do not shoot themselves or hang themselves, or fall in love, or deliver themselves of clever sayings every minute. They spend most of their time eating, drinking, running after women or men, talking nonsense. It is therefore necessary that this should be shown on stage. A play ought to be written in which people should come and go, dine, talk of the weather or play cards, not because the author wants it but because that is what happens in real life. Life on the stage should be as it really is, and the people, too, should be as they are and not on stilts.[1]

Although Chekhov was considerably influenced by Zola, his own poetic genius could not accept the Frenchman's exact bookkeeping of the facts. The same passion for objectivity and clinical analysis of the human animal which gives Chekhov so much of his strength feeds the work of Harold Pinter, who uses the conventions of Naturalism to go beyond them and chart mankind's evolving sense of its own boundaries.

Pinter, like Chekhov, has a distrust of simplifications. "I'm against all propaganda," he told Charles Marowitz in 1967, "even propaganda for life." His realism refuses to offer bromidic meanings or strained coherence to palliate forces beyond our comprehension. This uncompromising aesthetic took shape even before Pinter began writing plays. Commenting on the work of Samuel Beckett in a letter (1954), he said:

. . . I don't want philosophies, tracts, dogmas, creeds, ways
out, truths, answers, *nothing from the bargain basement.* He
[Beckett] is the most courageous, remorseless writer going
and the more he grinds my nose in the shit the more I am
grateful to him. He's not fucking me about, he's not leading
me up any garden, he's not slipping me any wink, he's not
flogging me a remedy or a path or a revelation or a basinful
of breadcrumbs, he's not selling me anything I don't want to
buy, he doesn't give a bollock whether I buy or not, he
hasn't got his hand over his heart. Well, I'll buy his goods,
hook, line, and sinker, because he leaves no stone unturned
and no maggot lonely. . . .[2]

Pinter's impulse is for a suprarealism which can offer a vision of life in its ambiguous entirety, a theatrical hypothesis
for an audience to entertain, in which all the facts are presented but never prejudged.

Man's dimensions of consciousness, his sense of a stable
position in the scheme of things, have changed in this century. Chekhov, for all his hard-headed analysis, wrote out of
a pastoral tradition to which the Russian gentry had become insensitive, one whose significance had been put into
question by a new urban order. The stage directions in *The
Cherry Orchard* (1904) are explicit:

*A road leads to Gayev's estate. On one side and some distance away is
a row of dark poplars, and it is there that the cherry orchard begins.
Farther away is seen a line of telegraph poles and beyond them, on the
horizon, the vague outlines of a large town, visible only in very good,
clear weather. . . .*[3]

Chekhov's lyricism—a counterpoint of words, gestures, and
sound—is always within the larger matrix of the country-
side. Pinter's world on the other hand is hermetically sealed
off from nature. His plays are urban fables in which no

poplars sway against the distant orchard, no wind under-scores human loneliness. Man's earthly garden, like the one in *The Caretaker*, is cluttered with lifeless, alien objects.

> DAVIES: Looks a bit thick.
> ASTON: Overgrown.
> DAVIES: What's that, a pond?
> ASTON: Yes.
> DAVIES: What you got, fish?
> ASTON: No. There isn't anything in there. *(Pause)*
> DAVIES: Where are you going to put your shed?
> ASTON *(turning)*: I'll have to clear the garden first.
> DAVIES: You'd need a tractor, man.

When Pinter invokes nature, it becomes a travesty, not only of pastoral simplicity, but of all those who would seek to recollect it in tranquillity. In *The Birthday Party*, Goldberg tries and fails to make an innocent bower of London's East End:

> When I was a youngster, of a Friday, I used to go for a walk down the canal with a girl who lived down my road. A beautiful girl. What a voice that bird had! A nightingale, my word of honor. Good? Pure? . . . We knew the meaning of respect. So I'd give her a peck and I'd bowl back home. I'd tip my hat to the toddlers, I'd give a helping hand to a couple of stray dogs, everything came natural. I can see it like yesterday. The sun falling behind the dog stadium. Ah!

This blarney is sensual, precise, and vacuous. Nature has become a cynical ploy, a marginal diversion, a moment of verbal muscle-flexing which balloons it to the proportions of myth (as in Hemingway), substituting an unreal self-con-sciousness for nature's inherent spontaneity.

In *The Sea Gull*, the lake is at first hidden by Treplev's wooden stage, an eclipse of nature by art significant for both Chekhov and his prototype of the young author. The play within the play is the embodiment of the Romantic Egotistical Sublime—a stillborn creation if there ever was one. Treplev demands an organic, natural background for something coldly intellectual. This contrast is wryly humorous; but when the curtain comes up on his little play, the lake asserts an undeniable power. Chekhov's stage directions indicate the primordial calm of the background: *"The curtain rises, revealing the view of the lake, with the moon above the horizon and its reflection in the water."* This setting is perfect for Treplev's theme of cosmic death and rebirth. He will create a new Eden, with its animal delights and verdant profusion transposed against a background which reminds the audience that nature still has something significant and sustaining to offer.

> NINA: The men, the lions, the eagles, the partridges, the antlered deer, the geese, the spiders, the silent fishes of the deep, starfishes and creatures unseen to the eye—in short all living things, all living things, having completed their mournful cycle, have been snuffed out. . . . In me the consciousness of men is merged with the instincts of animals: I remember it all, all, all, and live every single life anew in my own being.
>
> —*The Sea Gull* (I, i)

This speech is recalled by Nina in her last meeting with Treplev, and it stirs memories of a touching youthfulness and a talent never organized by a deeply felt vision of the world. Treplev kills himself—the lie of romantic egotism now apparent even to him.

Even if they escape ultimate destruction, the characters in Chekhov's plays tend to ossify in their rural surroundings. Vanya, the three sisters, and Arkadina reflect intellectual capacity turned flaccid. Astrov echoes Chekhov's sentiments:

> I love life as such—but our life, our everyday provincial life in Russia, I just can't endure. I despise it with all my soul. As for my own life, God knows I can find nothing good in it at all. You know, when you walk through a forest on a dark night and you see a small light gleaming in the distance you don't notice your tiredness, nor the darkness, nor the prickly branches lashing you in the face. . . .
>
> —*Uncle Vanya* (II, i)

In Chekhov's world, the blessings of nature are omnipresent, but the majority of mankind is unable to mirror the peacefulness and potential grace which surrounds it. In *The Cherry Orchard*, the Ranevsky family is forced from the family estate by their own class pretensions. The family exits to the thud of axes cutting the orchard, once the symbol of a luxuriant, safe world and now an accusation of their indifference to the environment which once sustained them. Even the final moments of *Uncle Vanya* reiterate this tension between the individual and nature. Sonia's sweet, vain longings are for an Eden whose visual correlative is outside her door.

> . . . We shall hear the angels, we shall see all the heavens covered with stars like diamonds, we shall see all earthly evil, all of our sufferings swept away by the grace which will fill the whole world, and our life will become peaceful, gentle, sweet as a caress. I believe it, I believe it. . . .

The watchman's tapping which fills the silence after Sonia's quiet pleading is the ironic Chekhovian smile. Sonia and Vanya are trapped; they cannot participate in nature's tranquillity. The boredom which pervades the life of Chekhov's characters has a palpable weight, an atmospheric pressure indicating their gradual withdrawal from the sustaining environment. One is, after all, never bored in nature as long as one can appreciate it.

Chekhov is writing, then, at the brink of a significant shift in man's attitude toward his place in the world. Chekhov's characters are both victims of nature's indifference and witnesses of its glory. A post-Darwinian ambivalence reverses former dramatic conventions of the pastoral. Country life in Russia does not bring the expected psychic release that Celia anticipates in *As You Like It* when she says, ". . . Now go we in content/To liberty and not to banishment." In Illyria or Arden, chaos is charmed into order. Disguise and misconception are games which can be happily played out apart from the world. Chekhov revises the idyllic image, evoking complexity from the stereotype of pastoral security, creating a world which offers no fixed meaning, but only fading shadows of coherence.

It is significant that Stanislavski, unable to capture the strong interior rhythms of Chekhov or understand the momentum created by the counterpoint between situation and environment, wanted to clutter the plays with real things. The effect was to glut the imagination, blurring the careful delineation of objects and sounds Chekhov had indicated in his stage directions. Stanislavski's *mise-en-scène* for *Uncle Vanya* is indicative:

> The play starts in darkness; an August evening. The dim light of a lantern set on top of a post; distant sounds of a

drunkard's song; distant howling of a dog; the croaking of frogs, the cry of a corn crake, the slow tolling of a distant church bell. All this helps the audience to get the feel of the sad and monotonous life of the characters. Flashes of lightning, faint rumblings of thunder in the distance. After the raising of the curtain a pause of ten seconds. After the pause, Yakov knocks, hammering in a nail (on the stage); having knocked the nail in, he busies himself on the stage, humming a tune.[4]

Chekhov's impressionistic technique demanded a more selectively focused *trompe-l'œil* effect, which tricked the audience into making thematic associations between characters and the sights and sounds surrounding them. The script reads simply: *"The sun has just set.* YAKOV *and other workmen are busy on the stage behind the lowered curtain; sounds of hammering and coughing."*

Chekhov's careful choice of key objects, from Treplev's stuffed sea gull to Vanya's elegant cravat, create a stagecraft oriented toward delicately accentuated things—a type of theater from which Stanislavski could generalize a theory of performing. As Eric Bentley has written, the Chekhovian method

> . . . requires two extraordinary gifts: the mastery of "petty" realistic material and the ability to go beyond sheer *Sachlichkeit*—materiality, factuality—to imagination and thought. . . . Now, the whole Stanislavski school of acting and directing is testimony that Chekhov was successfully *sachlich*—that is, not only accurate, but significantly precise, concrete, ironic. . . . The art by which a special importance is imparted to everyday objects is familiar enough in fiction; on stage, Chekhov is one of its few masters. . . .[5]

The breaking string, no matter how nonnaturalistic a sound, has a human focus and pertinence; the shimmering lake (*The Sea Gull*), the orchard flecked with May morning frost (*The Cherry Orchard*) still uphold man as the measure of his environment, implying a kind of proportion to reality which lends humanity to objects clearly nonhuman. In contrast, the object world in Pinter is never so certain; it offers no sounds of general discord and comment—like the breaking string. Nature allows no solace. His characters represent a modern consciousness wholly abstracted from its environment. The language, precise and sensual, tantalizes our sense of the real, only to disappear into the dynamics of the momentary situation. Max recalls a present to his wife in *The Homecoming*:

> . . . I said to her, Jessie, I think our ship is going to come home, I'm going to treat you to a couple of items, I'm going to buy you a dress in pale corded blue silk, heavily encrusted in pearls, and for casual wear, a pair of pantaloons in lilac flowered taffeta. Then I gave her a drop of cherry brandy.

Language, however, cannot isolate the past, and neither can memory. Chekhov hints at this in *The Three Sisters*. Olga's first words show the limitations of the human imagination, trying to control facts which are irretrievable: "It's exactly a year ago Father died, isn't it?" The finality of the statement is mocked by the rhetorical question. In the same way, Max's childhood is never as clear as his memory urges it to be.

> Our father! I remember him. Don't worry. You kid yourself. He used to come over to me and look down at me. My old man did. He'd bend right over me, then he'd pick me up. I was only that big. Then he'd dandle me. Give me the bottle.

Wipe me clean. Give me a smile. Pat me on the bum. Pass me around, pass me from hand to hand. Toss me up in the air. Catch me coming down. I remember my father.

The language seems specific, but behind Max's ferocious certainty is a world of shadows. He doesn't remember anything.

Pinter is obsessed by the arbitrary boundaries man makes for himself: the walls constructed of concrete, of language, of philosophy, which protect him from a capricious reality. In one of his early plays, *The Dwarfs* (1960), Pinter states what he later showed:

> LEN: The rooms we live in . . . open and shut. . . . Can't you see? They change shape at their own will. I wouldn't grumble if only they would keep to some consistency. But they don't. And I can't tell the limits, the boundaries which I've been led to believe are natural. . . .

In *The Birthday Party*, the house which has protected Stanley is turned into a menacing jungle. Pinter's attempts to transform the room are crude but effective. He throws the set into darkness during a game of blindman's buff, with a pursuer's flashlight scanning the room. The solidity evaporates. Objects become massive specters in the dark, threatening to overwhelm the guests. The light shines on the objects, assuring us that they exist, but they seem less than real. The walls protecting Stanley now incarcerate him, as McCann forces a flashlight into his face until his solidity and reason vaporize. When Stanley is taken away, the room comes back to "normal," only to expand again into uncertainty with the final dialogue:

> MEG: I was the belle of the ball.

PETEY: Were you? [. . .]
MEG: Oh, it's true . . . I was . . . *Pause.* . . . I know I was.

It is in *The Homecoming* that Pinter is able to achieve his most subtle interplay of naturalistic fact and a disturbingly fluid reality. Max's living room seems as logical as the human situation within it seems improbable. The stage has been stripped of excess, lacking the jumbled and claustrophobic qualities of *The Caretaker* or the nonchalant untidiness of the seaside boardinghouse of *The Birthday Party.* The set of *The Homecoming* consists of a mammoth arch, chairs, tables, the back wall broken through to expose a long staircase. The professor-son makes sure we, as well as his wife, Ruth, realize this is a controlled environment.

What do you think of the room? Big isn't it? It's a big house. I mean, it's a fine room, don't you think? Actually there was a wall, across there . . . with a door. We knocked it down . . . years ago . . . to make an open living area. The structure wasn't affected, you see. . . .

The room seems certain to the eye, filled with a steel-gray light as solid and reassuring as a Vermeer painting. It is immediately recognizable; the objects coax the audience into a comfortable acceptance. Both the surroundings and the characters appear mundane on stage. But that response is betrayed; the action uncovers elusive truths of sexual fantasy, lust, and impotence. As the play gathers momentum, the audience discovers—without Pinter forcing it—that the room has lost its apparent solidity. The stairway, covered by that monumental arch, takes on an unnatural, seductive, phallic length—an almost sexual potency.

Whereas Stanislavski developed the illusionistic "fourth wall" to give *The Sea Gull* the shock of reality, Pinter pushes against naturalistic stage conventions for his theatrical surprises. Sam, Max's aging brother, passing out, proclaims in his last breath that Max's deceased wife committed adultery in the back seat of his cab while he drove. A plot-point is wrapped up; something is explained. But *The Homecoming* is not a play in which the dead are carted off. The dialogue is Pinter at his best, mocking the "realistic" demands of a theater which hides man's most insensitive instincts.

> MAX: What's he done? Dropped dead?
> LENNY: Yes.
> MAX: A corpse? A corpse on my floor? Get him out of here!
>   Clear him out of here!
> JOEY *bends over* SAM.
> JOEY: He's not dead.
> LENNY: He probably was dead, for about thirty seconds.
> MAX: He's not even dead.

The action goes on around the body. No blackouts. No fine sentiment. People faint in subways or die, other people pass them by or give them a nudge of the boot to make sure they're still breathing. Pinter lets reality comment on itself, never pointing a finger.

In Chekhov's world, the language comments on an environment which demands answers, resolved careers. In all his plays, there are voices that speak of happiness, that yearn for a better world.

> OLGA: . . . But our sufferings may mean happiness for the people who come after us. . . . There'll be a time when peace and happiness reign in the world, and then we shall be remembered kindly and blessed. . . .

Olga, like her sisters, waits for a sign from nature (". . . Maybe if we wait a little longer we shall find out why we live, why we suffer. . . ."). Chekhov's world-view demanded both skepticism and hope:

> The best [classical writers] are realists and depict life as it is, because every line is permeated, as with a juice, by a conspicuousness of an aim; you feel in addition to life as it is life as it should be. . . . But what about us? We depict life as it is but we refuse to go a step further. We have neither near nor remote aims and our souls are as flat and bare as a billiard table. We have no politics, we do not believe in revolution, we deny the existence of God, we are not afraid of ghosts. . . . But he who wants nothing, hopes for nothing, and fears nothing cannot be an artist.[6]

Chekhov chronicles an existential stalemate, a problematic condition rather than a proposed answer. Yet there still remains the comforting solidity of possessions. Even though Lyuba Ranevsky loses her estate, the audience understands when she says, ". . . My dear bookcase! (*Kisses bookcase*) My own little table!" While symbols often emerge out of the dynamics of Chekhov's dramatic situations (Solyony's hands in *The Three Sisters*, the stuffed sea gull, etc.), there is a logic in their use which, while attesting to the randomness of experience, confesses a comforting sense of artistic order. The object world of Chekhov's plays never imposes itself on the experience of the characters as much as on their imagination. In Pinter, objects and gestures take on a physical potency which illustrates a mute isolation between man and object. Max swings his cane with a memory of sexual strength. Ruth weaves a mosaic of sensual innuendo, turning a glass of water into a throbbing organ:

RUTH: Have a sip. Go on. Have a sip from my glass. *He is still.* Sit on my lap. Take a long cool sip. *She pats her lap.*

Pause. She stands, moves to him with the glass. Put your head
back and open your mouth.

LENNY: Take that glass away from me.

RUTH: Lie on the floor. Go on. I'll pour it down your throat.

LENNY: What are you doing, making me some kind of pro-
posal?

Lenny has tried to overwhelm her with tales of violence
and sexual conquest. Ruth, however, by turning an object
into a threatening invitation, mocks our faith in the neu-
trality of material things. She offers, one might say, an
object lesson on the limitations of Man's sensory perception.

Look at me. I . . . move my leg. That's all it is. But I wear
. . . underwear . . . which moves with me . . . it . . .
captures your attention. Perhaps you misinterpret. The action is simple. It's a leg . . . moving. My lips move. Why
don't you restrict . . . your observations to that? Perhaps
the fact that they move is more significant . . . than the
words which come through them. You must bear that . . .
possibility . . . in mind.

Pinter's characters no longer cling to a wistful faith in
cosmic coherence. They have been permanently cut adrift
from their surroundings. They do not speak of hope or happiness; they simply want to survive from moment to moment. Chekhov explored the substance of man's life eroding
through time, but Pinter does something else with that dimension. All of Chekhov's characters come from a definable
past, and their futures, no matter how bleak, can be
charted. Irena will teach; Nina will act in the provinces;
Gaev will take a job as a bank clerk. The language of Chekhov's plays at their most poignant moments is heightened
by the future tense, by what will be. Futurity, like the "pa-

thetic fallacy" of seeing nature responding to man, implies a relationship to the world, a chronological order, a sense of the mind's evolutionary development. Pinter's language shows memory as a tractable tool, deceiving with seductive clarity. Memory holds no salvation and no value. Man can only live in an anxious, protracted present.

All Pinter's dramatic devices—the stylized speech, the weighted silences, the careful groupings—stress and heighten the moment. Pinter's drama moves where Nathalie Sarraute maintains the "new novel" must go: ". . . some precise dramatic action shown in slow motion . . . where time was no longer the time of real life, but a hugely amplified present. . . ."[7]

Pinter finds the language of music the easiest way to describe his own understanding of his plays. Like Chekhov, he orchestrates an elaborate composition of gestures, words, and pauses within the flexible unit of the room. Chekhov had already used the pause with moving dramatic and psychological insight. Lyuba and Gaev's last moment before leaving the estate is made more touching by being beyond words. If Pinter's plays seem to lack the rich tonality of Chekhov's works, it is because, in his view, nature gives us back no image of ourselves, and words, no matter how sensuous, are finally imprecise. The actor works in a smaller, more tightly controlled area of improvisation.

> I am very conscious of rhythm. It's got to happen [snapping his fingers] just like that, or it's wrong. I'm also interested in pitch. . . . I remember when we did *The Collection* Off-Broadway a few years ago, there was an American actor who was in big trouble with his part. I told him instead of trying to find reasons for his characterization, "Why don't you read the part and pay attention to the stress of the

words." He did it, and he was fine. The point is the stresses tell you what the meaning is. Saying it up or down can change the whole meaning. It has to be just right.

—PINTER, in a conversation

Silence becomes a more active factor in modern life; the past has blurred and the future is unknowable. Silence is a realistic device, as well as a symbol of cosmic indifference. As George Steiner has pointed out in *Language and Silence*: ". . . [when] language simply ceases, and the motion of the spirit gives no further outward manifestations of its being, the poet enters into silence. Here the word borders not on radiance or music, but on night."

Pinter, like Chekhov, uncovers a subterranean music. The difference in their techniques reflects the difference in evolving realistic appraisals of the world. If Pinter's world seems a smaller, grayer canvas, it is not a limitation of craft, but of the modern world—which leaves man with less faith in his mind, more fearful of the dehumanizing forces outside it.

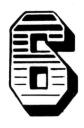

Joe Orton:
Artist of
the Outrageous

PRENTICE: I'm a rationalist.
RANCE: You can't be a rationalist in an
  irrational world. It isn't rational.

  —JOE ORTON, *What the Butler Saw* (1969)

With madness, as with vomit, it's the
passer-by who receives the
inconvenience. . . .

  —JOE ORTON, *The Erpingham Camp* (1966)

Joe Orton was the comedian of the dark side of the contemporary soul: the vituperative anti-Christ, isolated by his anarchist rage and cynical in his desolation. At the age of thirty-four, Orton was bludgeoned to death in his sleep by his roommate. This macabre demise is the kind of madness

Orton savored in his farces. Bloody, perverse, ostensibly mo-
tiveless—Orton's murder would have seemed to him the
final outrage: an event as mysterious, gratuitous, and
amoral as his birth.

Orton gives a logic and an emotional truth to the perverse in experience. In his early plays—*The Ruffian on the
Stair* (1964), *Entertaining Mr. Sloane* (1964)—the outrageous
springs from an apparent realism. Society's mores are always butting heads with fatuous catastrophe. (As one prissy
onlooker observes in the bedlam of Orton's *What the Butler
Saw*: "Two young people—one mad and one sexually insatiable—both naked—are roaming this house. At all costs we
must prevent a collision.") In Orton's plays, madness and
reason inevitably collide. There is a humanity behind this,
an attempt to make an audience learn from its outcasts and
understand that every man is lost, bound together in communal madness. Orton tries to establish through theater the
new channels of feeling R. D. Laing has postulated in psychology:

> . . . When will the charade turn to carnival? Saints may
> still be kissing lepers. It is high time lepers kissed the
> saints. . . .[1]

Orton's plays offend in order to instruct and heal; they
shatter the easy divisions of we and they, the good and the
bad, the just and the unjust.

INTERVIEWER: It's interesting how in *Loot* a number of people are offended in that so much of the action is centered
around a coffin.
ORTON: I never understand why, because if you're abso-
lutely practical—and I hope I am—a coffin is only a box.
One calls it a coffin and once you've called it a coffin it immediately has all sorts of implications. In *Entertaining Mr.*

Sloane, I wrote about a man who was interested in boys and liked having sex with boys. I wanted him to be played as if he was the most ordinary man in the world, and not as if the moment you wanted sex with boys you had to put on earrings and scent. This is very bad. . . . It's compartmentalization again. Audiences love it, of course, because they're safe. . . . What I wanted to do in *Sloane* was break down all the sexual compartments people have. . . .[2]

Orton's wit exposes the arrogance behind conventional wisdom. In *The Erpingham Camp*, a priest initiates an eager new flunky at a holiday resort into the corporate structure. He hands the young man a Bible: "Take God's blessing with you, my son. And remember always to keep the little book I gave you. The words are obscure but the pictures will keep you from harm." Orton preys on those institutions which enforce a pious authority and an emotional rigidity: the Church ("It's life that defeats the Christian Church. She's always been able to deal with death"), the State ("You're at liberty to answer your own doorbell, miss. That is how we tell whether or not we live in a free country").

The outrageous can become shrill and extreme in its hate; but Orton's humor is deliciously double-edged in skewering both victim and victimizer. Orton denies synthetic emotions. In *The Ruffian on the Stair*, Mike, a petty thief, lives with Joyce, a whore who is his "wife." An intruder, Wilson, seeks revenge for the hit-and-run killing of his brother. Mike shoots Wilson, ostensibly for "sleeping" with Joyce. A stray bullet breaks the goldfish bowl.

JOYCE: They're dead. Poor things. And I reared them so carefully. And while all this was going on they died.
MIKE: Sit down. I'll fetch the police. This has been a crime of passion. They'll understand. They have wives and goldfish of their own.

(JOYCE *is too heartbroken to answer. She buries her face in* MIKE'*s shoulder. He holds her close. Curtain*)

Orton's couple is left in squalid yet hilarious isolation. The value of human life is less than that of a goldfish. Orton's objectivity will not allow sentimentality even among the most intimate social rituals, such as a funeral. In *Loot* (1967), the son of the deceased refuses the ex-nurse's suggestion to pay his respects to the dead.

> FAY: What excuse do you give?
> HAL: It would upset me.
> FAY: That's exactly what a funeral is meant to do.

From Orton's perspective, the outrageous is in the eyes of the beholder. In *Loot*, Hal, the homosexual son, contemplates burying his mother nude in order to put his stolen money in her coffin, and plots with the ex-nurse about how she'll marry his father to get the inheritance:

> HAL: Bury her naked? My own Mum? *(He goes to the mirror and combs his hair)* It's a Freudian nightmare.
> DENNIS: I won't disagree.
> HAL: Aren't we committing some kind of unforgivable sin?
> DENNIS: Only if you're Catholic.

In Orton's plays, sexuality is as ordinary as mashed potatoes. Hal admits his predilection for boys; the nurse scolds him:

> FAY: Most people of any influence will ignore you. You'll be forced to associate with young men like yourself. Does that prospect please you?
> HAL: I'm not sure.

FAY: Well, hesitation is something to be going on with. We can build on that. What will you do when you're old?

HAL: I shall die.

FAY: I see you're determined to run the gamut of all experience.

Sexual appetite is its own justification. In *Entertaining Mr. Sloane*, a brother and sister both have sexual designs on a boarder, Sloane, who proceeds to kill their father. They decide, finally, to share him for their pleasure rather than turn him over to the police. Ed and Kath argue over him with the righteousness of conventional indignation:

KATH: I gave him everything. . . . What more could he want?

ED: Freedom.

KATH: He's free with me.

ED: You're immoral.

KATH: He's clean-living by nature; that's every man's right.

Orton disguises himself as an immoralist in order to re-examine the morality of the age. Orton's outrageousness works against conventional response. He puts his anger within a theatrical structure whose framework gives the stage actions humor as well as menace. The melodramatic conventions of modern "serious theater" (and their implications) become his targets as well as his dramatic devices. The Intruder and the Unknown are part of a melodramatic pattern whose comfortable tension Orton inverts. In *The Ruffian on the Stair*, the "villain," Wilson, enters an emotional waste land instead of a bower of domestic tranquillity. He is neither a frothing imbecile nor a chest-thumping rapist. He has, in fact, an eye for the men:

I'm a Gents hairdresser. Qualified. My dad has a business. Just a couple of chairs. I've clipped some notable heads in my time. Mostly professional men. Though we had an amateur street musician in a few weeks ago. We gave him satisfaction, I believe.

When Wilson is gunned down, Orton uses the moment to mock the tidy emotional clarity of melodrama. Instead of the *status quo* being restored, ignorance is compounded:

> WILSON: He's shot me. My will is in my overcoat pocket. My address in my pocket diary. Remember, will you?
> JOYCE *(to* MIKE*)*: What've you done?
> WILSON: He took it serious. How charming. *(He coughs, blood spurts from his mouth)* He's a bit of a nutter if you ask me. Am I dying? I think . . . oh . . .
> JOYCE: He's fainted.

Death clarifies nothing. In the excess of stage emotion, there need not be dignity. The gush of blood from Wilson's mouth impresses Joyce only enough to make her venture that he has passed out. The brutality of life, in Orton's eyes, comes from mankind's unwillingness to see what it has created. The outrageous is a means of denying this process of evasion. At the conclusion of *Loot*, with the money safe, the nurse, the son, and his boy friend happily free of the law, Orton concludes with a joke on the forced, bland harmony of conventional farce:

> HAL *(to* DENNIS*)*: You can kip here, baby. Plenty of room now. Bring your bags over tonight.
> FAY: When Dennis and I are married we'd have to move out.
> HAL: Why?
> FAY: People would talk. We must keep up appearances.
> *(Curtain)*

The conclusions of boulevard farce are illusions which hide a disturbing truth. Orton's farces rejuvenate techniques of melodrama within farce while commenting on them. In *What the Butler Saw*, the psychiatrist inspector, Dr. Rance, tries to explain the situation to the wife of the head of the clinic:

> RANCE: . . . Your husband has made away with his secretary!
> MRS. PRENTICE: Isn't that a little melodramatic, Doctor?
> RANCE: Lunatics are melodramatic. . . .

By extending the complexities of plot and psychological reversals to the extremes of farce, Orton finds a theatrical format whose size and tone match the pseudosanity he wants to expose.

I

> JOYCE: . . . The number of humiliating
> admissions I've made. You'd think it would
> draw me closer to somebody. But it doesn't.
>
> —JOE ORTON, *The Ruffian on the Stair*

Farce is thought of as a bourgeois fun machine in which the people of the stage world try frantically (and hopelessly) to make connections with one another. The frenetic rhythms of farce, the confusion of identity, and the passionate actions based on misunderstanding offer a precise theatrical correlative to Orton's view of social insanity. In farce, people are pushed out of their minds, propelled by the momentum of circumstances, not free will. As the impetus increases, humanity disintegrates before our eyes. People bounce off one another, only to rebound in their stupor and try again. They speak in earnest; but their private despair is swept away by the acceleration of events. The farce structure, once so patently artificial, captures the tempo and confusion of modern living. As R. D. Laing points out:

> When the ultimate basis of our world is in question, we run to different holes in the ground, we scurry into roles, statuses, identities, interpersonal relations. . . . Each [person] sometimes sees the same fragment of the whole situation differently; often our concern is with different presentations of the original catastrophe.[3]

Boulevard farce takes place amid velours curtains and *chaises longues*. It is a confident form, glorifying in the world's solidity. Boulevard farce wears a debonair smile, is worldly-wise, and indifferent to the vagaries of the universe. Its laughter does not acknowledge pain, only a world of jaded wealth, sweaty *affaires*, passions conceived in boredom, and a fascination with the gadgets and games of the *nouveaux riches*. No matter how tortuous the convolutions of plot, the people in boulevard farce manage to escape destruction. They are a little embarrassed perhaps, or momentarily foiled, but never vanquished by their ignorance. Boulevard farce underscores the middle-class daydreams of coherence —a world where events have their order and life's blows turn out to be benign.

Orton is a modern *farceur* who sees life as precarious. He blasts the soft assumptions of boulevard entertainment while mastering its mechanism for mayhem. Orton takes farce past Georges Feydeau. He moves the laughter out of the parlor and puts it in a mortuary (*Loot*) and a psychiatric clinic (*What the Butler Saw*). The predicaments of the old farce (the secret rendezvous, the hidden lover, the foolproof plan) have the potential, but not the conviction, of tragedy. In Orton's farces, the only destiny is ambiguous survival.

Orton brings farce back to the world of death, destruction, and betrayal that boulevard laughter tries to gloss over in its confidence. Orton's humor confronts life instead of escaping from it. Where Feydeau avoids high seriousness in his fun, Orton finds a despair in laughter which chronicles the psychic death in life. Orton's world offers no safety to its characters, only violent adjustments—as random and urgent as the predicaments of farce. At the end of *Loot*, the police inspector arrests the wrong man: Mr. McLeavy, the recent widower and father of the robber. As McLeavy is carted off to jail, he screams a testimony. His righteous indignation confuses morality with Catholic superstition. He exits, saying, "I'm innocent. I'm innocent. Oh, what a terrible thing to happen to a man who's been kissed by the Pope."

Farce is the most anarchic stage form. Characters are motivated not by deep, rational understanding or insight but by intuition and the vagaries of the moment. For Orton, farce is ideally suited to his purpose of demythologizing man's rational powers. In *Entertaining Mr. Sloane*, Sloane confesses that he killed a man: "I had no motive." In farce, this intellectual ambivalence is carried to extremes. It is the genre's power that the characters who vault out of closets or dash under beds at superhuman speeds do so in the name of the most primitive impulses. Most types of theater emphasize man's rationality; farce emphasizes his animality. *Loot*

is Orton's first full-fledged farce. The play exudes a joyous
literary liberation and a sense of control. It is as if—having
found the form for his talent—Orton wanted to topple
every boundary. The deceased receives a memorial wreath
from the Friends of Bingo. Fay, the nurse, who at the age of
twenty-eight has already outlived and outwitted seven hus-
bands, urges the widower, Mr. McLeavy, to marry her. "Go
ahead," she says. "Ask me to marry you. I've no intention of
refusing. On your knees. I'm a great believer in traditional
positions." Unlike boulevard farce where the language is as
mundane as the people, Orton's words are as unpredictable
and unnerving as his characters' morality.

In farce, the body is transformed by anarchy's energy.
Man no longer stands quite erect, but is changed by farce
into an acrobatic and contorted machine. The body undergoes the gamut of pulverizing experiences. In *Loot*, for instance, the son, Hal, dumps his mother's corpse in a closet
to make room for the stolen money in the coffin. The humiliation is compounded when they drag her out to undress
her in order to do away with any evidence:

FAY: Are you committed to having her teeth removed?
HAL: Yes. . . . *(He holds up her teeth)* . . . These are good
teeth. Are they the National Health?
FAY: No. She bought them out of her winnings. She had
some good evenings at the table last year.

When they are transferring the body from the closet, an
eye falls out. The culprits scramble on their hands and
knees in search of it; not to preserve the wholeness of the
corpse, but to eliminate the evidence. The detective, Truscott, discovers it; but, typical of Orton's vision of inhuman-

ity, Truscott has difficulty identifying the part of the human anatomy. The stage direction reads: ". . . *He holds it to the light in order to get a better view. Puzzled. He sniffs at it. He holds it close to his ear. He rattles it. He takes out a pocket magnifying glass and stares hard at it. . . .*"

Whereas *Loot* and *The Erpingham Camp* explore farce as anarchy, *What the Butler Saw*, written in 1967, extends the genre to a vision of total madness. Orton's most profound and most skillful play integrates his wit with masterful contortions of plot. *What the Butler Saw* builds an internal pressure and mental confusion which simulate the despair behind neurosis. Dr. Prentice, a psychiatrist, is sneakily attempting to undress his new secretary under the ruse of a medical checkup. Enter Mrs. Prentice, a nymphomaniac who loathes her husband. She confesses to being blackmailed by the page boy at a local hotel for indiscretions with him. Dr. Prentice tries to hide his seminude secretary from his wife. The page boy arrives with photographs of Mrs. Prentice in the act. He gets mixed up in the confusion. The girl must dress in his page-boy costume to escape. The boy must wear a wig and skirt to go unnoticed. Added to the hysteria of this scramble, the psychiatrist inspector, Dr. Rance, comes to look over the clinic and arrives at the conclusion that Dr. Prentice is sicker than anyone under his care.

This is the schizophrenic predicament as R. D. Laing has described it. Prentice too "does not know where he is or where he is going. He cannot get anywhere however hard he tries. . . . The future is the result of the present, the present is the result of the past and the past is unalterable." [4] Farce makes us forget everything but the manic needs of the moment. The audience sees the logic in Dr.

Prentice's cover-ups; the stage characters do not. He is not really mad; but the stage characters read madness into his every practical, private response. This begins to erode his sense of sanity. Dr. Prentice, for instance, writes letters to *The Guardian*. From this, his wife and Dr. Rance deduce neurosis.

> MRS. PRENTICE: Are you ashamed of the fact that you write to strange men?
> PRENTICE: There's nothing furtive in my relationship with the editor of *The Guardian*. . . .

All the characters in *What the Butler Saw* are numbed and dizzied by the speed of experience. They lose any sense of where and who they are. Mrs. Prentice, a confessed nymphomaniac, sees her dream come true. The reality is too much. After witnessing the scurry of seminude bodies, she collapses, screaming, "Doctor, Doctor! The world is full of naked men running in all directions." Sexual identities are not only physically confused, but emotionally uncertain. Geraldine, the secretary dressed as a page boy, is interrogated by Dr. Rance:

> RANCE: . . . Do you think yourself a girl?
> GERALDINE: No.
> RANCE: Why not?
> GERALDINE: I'm a boy.
> RANCE *(kindly)*: Do you have the evidence about you?
> GERALDINE *(her eyes flashing an appeal to* DR. PRENTICE*)*: I must be a boy. I like girls.

Events spiral out of control; each person sees them from his own angle. Farce never allows anyone on stage to see the same thing. This leads to a state of complete emotional polarization. Dr. Prentice wants to commit Dr. Rance, whose actions seem preposterous to him; and Dr. Rance wants to commit Dr. Prentice. There is no shared experience; each is struggling to preserve his sanity—not through understanding but by eliminating the source of tension.

PRENTICE *(waving his gun)*: . . . I'm going to certify you.
RANCE *(quietly, with dignity)*: No, I am going to certify you.
PRENTICE: I have the weapon. You have the choice. What is it to be? Either madness or death?
RANCE: Neither of your alternatives would enable me to continue to be employed by Her Majesty's Government.
PRENTICE: That isn't true. The higher reaches of the civil service are recruited entirely from corpses or madmen. Press the alarm!

Orton's image following this speech is stunning. When the alarm is pulled, "grilles" come down over every door, and sirens sound. Caged, furious, and arrogant in its denial of madness, the stage world becomes such a nightmare that the people in it can justifiably ask assurances of their existence. The page boy "crawls, almost fainting" to a chair.

NICK: What about me, sir? I'm not mad.
RANCE *(with a smile)*: You're not human.
NICK: I can't be an hallucination. *(He points to his bleeding shoulder)* Look at this wound. That's real.
RANCE: It appears to be.
NICK: If the pain is real I must be real.
RANCE: I'd rather not get involved in metaphysical speculations.

II

There is a social truth behind farce's mechanics which connects the stage madness to the schizophrenic hysteria of contemporary life. Orton's genius is in making this connection. In farce, the characters become hilariously powerless in the face of events. Orton sees this not simply as the condition of fun, but of life. *What the Butler Saw* concludes with most of the characters stripped to their underwear by the vagaries of events. "Let us put on our clothes and face the world," says Dr. Rance. But in this modern evocation of Adam and the "fortunate fall," innocence, truth, and energy have been outlandishly betrayed. Orton's final stage direction leaves the audience with a devastating self-image: *"They pick up their clothes and weary, bleeding, drugged and drunk, climb the rope ladder into the blazing light."*

Farce makes a shell game of experience: now you see it, now you don't. The audience is given an omniscience the characters never have. As the plot balloons, there is no way to control the confusions. The effect is to create a sense of powerlessness in the stage world which is at the root of neurosis in the real one. R. D. Laing has described the schizophrenic in terms that could apply to any Orton farce character:

> In his life situation the person comes to feel that he is in an untenable position. He cannot make a move, or make no move, without being beset by contradictory and paradoxical pressures and demands, pushes and pulls, both internally from himself and externally from those around him. He is, as it were, in a position of checkmate.[5]

Under these pressures man turns into himself as a tactic

of evasion. He becomes mad to avoid the tensions of a ruthless world. In *Loot*, the predicament is dramatized when Truscott arrests Mr. McLeavy. The individual is trammeled by irresponsible authority:

McLEAVY: I want to see someone in authority.
TRUSCOTT: I am an authority. You can see me.
McLEAVY: Someone higher.
TRUSCOTT: You can see whoever you like providing you convince me first that you're justified in seeing them.

The nightmare of this injustice is built into the logic of the system of farce, just as it is built into the system of government. Confusion, ignorance, and insanity reign under the disguise of propriety:

McLEAVY: You're mad.
TRUSCOTT: Nonsense. I had a checkup only yesterday. Our medical officer assured me that I was quite sane.
McLEAVY: I'm innocent. *(A little unsure of himself, the beginning of panic)* Doesn't that mean anything to you?

Orton shows how fragile the illusion of sanity is; and how, out of ignorance, people invoke their mental health. Mr. McLeavy cannot make his case understood; Truscott parries his requests with words on a totally different moral wave length. For McLeavy, the next step is madness. He knows the truth but is shown to be wrong by a man to whom truth and humanity have never mattered. McLeavy screams on stage out of fear of his impending powerlessness, just as Bobby Seale, bound and gagged in the Chicago conspiracy trial, yelled at Judge Hoffman. Seale had dismissed his lawyer in order to defend himself. The lawyer, William

Kunstler, had made this known to the judge; but the judge would not recognize the fact. The court dialogue has the painful truth of an Orton farce:

> THE COURT: Mr. Seale and Mr. Kunstler, your lawyer, I must admonish you that such outbursts are considered by the Court to be contemptuous, contumacious, and will be dealt with appropriately in the future.
> MR. KUNSTLER: Your Honor, the defendant was trying to defend himself, and I have already indicated my—
> THE COURT: The defendant was not defending himself.
> MR. SEALE: I was too defending myself. Any time anybody gives me the wrong symbol in the courtroom is deliberately—
> THE COURT: He is not addressing me with authority—
> MR. SEALE:—distorting and putting it on the record.
> THE COURT: Instruct that man to keep quiet.
> MR. SEALE: I want to defend myself. . . . No siree, I am not going to sit here and get that on the record. I am going to at least let it be known . . . that this man is erroneously representing symbols directly related to the party of which I am chairman.[6]

What the Butler Saw exposes the social madness which America now experiences. The visible tension in farce has become the pattern of our society. As in Orton's play, the nation has reached a momentum over Vietnam where truth no longer matters:

> GERALDINE: I'm not a patient. I'm telling the truth.
> RANCE: It's much too late to tell the truth.

Our political leaders, like Dr. Rance in *What the Butler Saw*, are faced with their own brutality. Their evasion of this inhumanity is made in the name of "sanity" which they call pragmatism:

MRS. PRENTICE: Is this real blood?

RANCE: No.

MRS. PRENTICE: Can you see it?

RANCE: Yes.

MRS. PRENTICE: Then what explanation is there?

RANCE: I'm a scientist. I state facts, I cannot be expected to provide explanations. Reject any para-normal phenomena. It's the only way to remain sane.

Spiro Agnew's impugning of the news media stems from the same psychotic impulse behind Dr. Rance's words: the attempt to restore "sanity" by ignoring the madness which has been created in the name of reason. Agnew is talking the language of censorship under the guise of moral indignation. He does not want the truth of Vietnam or the protest movement to be seen. He forces those who protest against madness into a state of frustration approaching insanity. Ultimately, they must ask what Orton's characters ask: are they real? Are the alternatives (in Dr. Prentice's words) madness or death? There seems to be no middle ground between what they know about the world and what authority wants them to believe. This problem of perception is a theme reiterated through Orton's work and borne out in America. Agnew, in his famous Harrisburg, Pennsylvania, speech, welcomed this dichotomy. His words are as insane as Dr. Rance's. He would feed the dementia. ". . . If in challenging peace demonstrators we polarize American people, I say it is time for positive polarization." The protector willingly becomes the victimizer. Agnew speaks with a vague, intense patriotism. Like Detective Truscott in *Loot*, Agnew's words hide him from the violence of his actions. Truscott asks Hal where he has stashed the money. Hal answers. Then Truscott kicks him violently:

TRUSCOTT: Don't lie to me!

HAL: I'm not lying! It's in the church!

TRUSCOTT *(shouting, knocking* HAL *to the floor)*: Under any other political system I'd have you on the floor in tears.

HAL *(crying)*: You've got me on the floor in tears.

Repression is not merely a political maneuver; it is a psychotic response for dealing with the unknown. The paranoia of the right wing is fed by its ignorance of the world. Agnew talks of "separating the protest leaders from our society—with no more regret than we should feel over discarding rotten apples from a barrel." The same violent arrogance and pseudosanity is reflected in Dr. Rance's righteous reaction to Dr. Prentice's "crime." Like the Nixon Administration, Dr. Rance has a barbaric conspiratorial view of the world which sees things that do not exist yet cannot interpret the physical facts in front of it:

RANCE: . . . Society must be made aware of the growing menace of pornography. The whole treacherous avant-garde movement will be exposed for what it is—an instrument for inciting the humanity and the state. . . .

The velocity of public life has the momentum of an Orton farce. Like Orton's stage characters, the public is unwittingly numbed by the experience. "I've been too long among the mad to know what sanity is," confesses Dr. Prentice, expressing a confusion of roles infecting our own society. President Nixon does not feel the shame of American massacres or see the nation's mortifying defeats in Vietnam when he talks of our "destiny," or when he maintains, "North Vietnam cannot defeat or humiliate the United States; only Americans can do that." The madness lies in his inability to see that the country he is destroying is the one he would defend.

Orton's farces make an audience confront the schizophrenic patterns of their lives, rather than evade them. By making a carnival of man's stupidity and superstition, by exposing the condition of social insanity, his plays hold out to an audience the possibility of humility and care. As a genre, farce has a power and insidious appeal which is becoming increasingly pertinent to our historical moment. Orton's plays, especially *What the Butler Saw*, pave a new way for playwrights to create dangerously with laughter in dangerous times. Orton's writing is a testament to what American society is just beginning to realize: reality is the ultimate outrage.

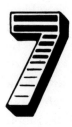

Jules Feiffer
and Sam Shepard:
Spectacles of Disintegration

In 1970, American society is panicked at the sight of its disintegration. Death haunts the communal imagination. The nation's self-deception in the Vietnam war and in its domestic law and order has turned its citizens into murderers. Abroad, we live out the humiliation and confusion of useless massacres like My Lai. Domestic frustrations build as the contradictions in the nation multiply and are not remedied. Guerrilla cadres blow up buildings; civil-rights workers and political dissidents are murdered or, as in the Chicago conspiracy trial, incarcerated and violently silenced. In the process, neither the victim nor the victimizer escapes without psychic wounds.

To be responsible in such a climate, our theater must be visionary. Like the society, the stage must forge new images —not only to revitalize the imaginative life of its audience but to attempt to give form to our incredible fragmentation and despair. Our theater rarely offers its audiences truly contemporary images. The society's sickness is beyond the finger-pointing and name-calling of protest theater, and too complex and gargantuan for an accessible naturalism. The oppressive sense of death and betrayal, the yearnings for purity and rebirth which fill the nation's dream life, take their most effective form in the mockery of grotesque fantasy. In this there is a denial of death, an attempt to push out the imaginative possibilities of the stage and the society. To succeed, such theater must be shocking, violent, and unpredictable. The characters may not be fleshed out with a weighty realism of the past. American life is marked by a profound shallowness, and such theatrical flatness is itself a comment on the erosion of personality in our age. Jules Feiffer's *The White House Murder Case* and Sam Shepard's *Operation Sidewinder* show the American theater grappling with sources of the nation's madness and spiritual displacement. Feiffer's satire deals with the process of moral decay in which a society becomes numb to its own homicide; Shepard's is a panorama of the waste land this self-deception creates and the frantic search by the society for new psychic imagery in order to survive it.

I

The government tries to anesthetize the public and itself from the pain of its failures. President Nixon asks the nation to lower its voice. Vice-President Agnew denies the integrity of public protest:

As for these deserters, malcontents, radicals, incendiaries, the civil and uncivil disobedients among our young, SDS,

PLP, Weathermen 1 and Weathermen 2, the Revolutionary Action Movement, the Yippies, Hippies, Yahoos, Black Panthers, lions and tigers alike—I would swap the whole damn zoo for a single platoon of the kind of young Americans I saw in Vietnam.

The White House Murder Case dramatizes this process of numbing by which both leaders and soldiers adapt to the inhumanity of their roles. It shows Americans dummying up a destiny on the battlefield and in the confines of a Cabinet meeting. The U.S. is now fighting "Chico" in Brazil. By accident, nerve gas has been dropped by Americans on American troops. The play follows both constituencies as they try to fictionalize their failures. The soldiers are extensions of the politicians. The GIs fight on the periphery of the White House room, the battles melding into the Cabinet meeting scenes. The soldiers are physically disintegrating from nerve gas; the politicians' disintegration is spiritual.

The soldiers, like the politicians, are fascinated by their "image." Duty substitutes for destiny. Their "image" is an anodyne for the brutality of their actions:

> CUTLER: The first thing you got to learn is how to take orders. The second thing you got to learn is how to look good. All your buddies are looking good. You don't want your buddies to see you not looking good. That's how you start. After a while it gets to be automatic. . . .

In the same way, *Realpolitik* glosses over the politician's self-deception. The commander of the U.S. Brazilian campaign, General Pratt, is called into the Cabinet. General Pratt is temporarily blinded and partially paralyzed by the nerve gas. He has no voice; his neck brace is miked. He is a hollow man, a walking echo chamber. The satiric encounter is an image of the nation's "leaders" and "warriors" brutalized beyond feeling.

> SWEENEY: On the basis of evidence in the field, can you draw any conclusions about the span of CB97 effectiveness?
> PRATT: My own conclusion is that there is a declining scale of effectiveness after six minutes. . . . It was no more than 50 per cent in terms of myself; I was blinded, paralyzed on the left side, suffered second-degree facial burns and damage to my voice.
> SWEENEY: I would rate that higher than 50 per cent.
> PRATT: I would agree, completely.

One way to control history is to make it up. Feiffer dramatizes this when the President's wife—a liberal critic of her husband's politics—is murdered in the Cabinet room. The Cabinet deals with this crisis as just another political pratfall. The politicians try to decide who did it and then, unable to reach a decision, how to rationalize it. Feiffer's Secretary of Defense summarizes a terrifying pattern which our nation has witnessed in the government's fabrications about the Gulf of Tonkin, My Lai, the *Pueblo* Incident:

> PARSON: So that's the question: Do we go on and let events push us around or do we use our initiative and take control of our destinies instead of vice versa?
> PRESIDENT: I'm sorry but I don't understand what you're saying.
> PARSON: My recommendation, Mr. President, is that the First Lady was assassinated by a suicide squad of Brazilian terrorists.

Both the politicians and the soldiers try to hold their
world together. The GI, wounded and disintegrating, imagines his companion as "Chico" and shoots him:

> WEEMS: We're all together, Buzz. You've got my hand!
> CUTLER: I don't want your faggot hand! You're not a man.
>   You're not an American. You're Chico!

The madness is not merely in the man but in the nature
of the conflict. Commenting on the massacres in Vietnam,
Robert J. Lifton wrote:

> In addition to the psychological principle that killing can
> relieve the fear of being killed, there is something else oper-
> ating here: the momentary illusion on the part of GIs that,
> by gunning down these figures now equated with the
> enemy, they were finally involved in a genuine "military ac-
> tion" in which their elusive adversaries were located, made
> to stand still, and annihilated: an illusion that they had
> finally put their world back in order.[1]

Feiffer satirizes the murkiness behind every Presidential
decision. The President makes a political deal with the
Postmaster General, who is his wife's confessed murderer,
and who threatens to admit his crime to the press, thus ru-
ining the President's chances for re-election. The President
calls his Cabinet together, and they achieve "unity" by
agreeing to his fabrication:

> PRESIDENT: As some of you may have heard, the First Lady
>   flew to Chicago last night for a short vacation. I learned
>   by phone that she has been taken seriously ill. The doc-
>   tors suspect food poisoning.
> OTHERS (*in chorus*) : Oh, I'm sorry, Mr. President.

The White House Murder Case shows us a world in which no historical event, no public image, no emotional relationship is authentic. The politicians do not see themselves as killers, yet their answer to the problems of society is destruction. Self-deception becomes the mechanism by which they hide the fear of rootlessness and stagnation—their own symbolic death—from themselves.

Feiffer's satire is more literary than theatrical. He embraces the grotesque but he does not extend it into a theatrical style. The horror of his satire results from witnessing the outrageous spring so logically from the conventional. The anxiety that such continual betrayals create within the nation inspire the apocalyptic fantasy of Sam Shepard's *Operation Sidewinder*. The fear of spiritual death, the cruelties of a faceless, omnipotent government, and the lack of any national purpose are the driving forces behind his epic adventure story. Shepard's theatricality uses the grotesque to evoke the frantic mood of contemporary America.

II

Operation Sidewinder begins with an image of strangulation. The lights come up on a desert. A mammoth snake, its eyes blinking like red beacons, is poised to strike. Two tourists— Honey and her husband, Dukie—stop to photograph the curiosity. While Dukie sets up his tripod, Honey gets too close to the snake. The snake leaps; she is caught in its powerful coil. Dukie photographs the event while barking orders to her, and then runs for help. The image sets the tone of the play: grotesque, horrific, and darkly comic. Things are out of joint, and people, surrounded by images of disintegration and death, are as numb to them as is Dukie, who is photographing the preposterous embrace. Shepard strings his play out in episodes which counterpoint the country rock music played by the Holy Modal Rounders. Each scene is like a panel in a medieval triptych (a small mystery which is clarified only after one experiences the entire event). The theatrical experience is deepened by the musical one, which, like print in medieval illuminated manuscripts, is for a modern audience an explicit but less familiar language than the stage image.

The characters react to death and the threat of it in an aloof, absurd way. Shepard's central figure, the Young Man, is waiting nervously for his car to be fixed at a desert garage. The car has a mysterious ailment—its lights blink uncontrollably. Dukie races in for help. The Young Man wants his car. The mechanic tries to calm Dukie down. The Young Man draws a gun and demands that the mechanic get on with the work. Dukie makes a panic-stricken move. The gun goes off, almost by surprise, and Dukie is dead. Seconds later, the mechanic is shot, and he somersaults backward in a parody of a gun-duel death.

The Young Man is obsessed with carrying out a crackpot, radical scheme to seize Air Force planes on the desert by dropping dope into a military reservoir. He is delivering guns for Mickey Free, the Indian renegade who will actually make the drop to his contact, an old prospector. Their meeting place is the spot where Honey has been attacked. She is still writhing with the snake. The prospector gabbles on to Honey as if he were daydreaming. He talks about the decay of the old mining towns, but not of her danger. The Young Man arrives but pays no attention to Honey. The prospector points her out to him. "She's got nothing to do with me," the Young Man says, handing over the gun and leaving. In order to survive, the Young Man cannot permit himself to feel for others. Death surrounds him and he acts as though his emotions were frozen.

The Air Force officers are introduced into *Operation Sidewinder* in an oblique, alcoholic discussion about hunting dogs. The military men are literally numb from drinking; they too are cut off from themselves and the world. They are debating remedies, not for society but for their animals. They talk about them as people to justify loving them, whereas the reverse process—dehumanizing people and describing them as pigs, dogs, freaks—makes it easier to justify killing humans:

> COLONEL WARNER: Trouble with that bitch, you just didn't get her out in the world enough, Henry. A young bitch like that's gotta come in contact with a whole lotta people and noise. Otherwise, you'll just never get her cured.

Everyone is struggling to survive. Mickey Free, the half-breed, cuts Honey loose from the snake, keeping the gigantic head for himself. The Young Man enters with the dope and the final plans. Again he blocks out Honey's predicament: "I see you're free now. Why don't you split?" But the irony, reiterated continually through the play, is that because of individual obsessions (means of psychically sidestepping death) no one is free. Mickey Free has sold his Indian birthright in order to survive. He has killed his own tribesmen; he has led the white man to the land which is now the military installation he is plotting to destroy. The Young Man makes the final arrangements. Mickey Free leaves. The Young Man is left alone with Honey and the severed body of the snake. He starts to shoot up, but he has no belt. He tries using the snake's massive coil. The extent of his despair is measured by the exaggeration of that gesture. In this barren terrain, anything that will give life or alleviate the sense of decay is acceptable. A song makes the point:

> It doesn't matter what you try it's all about take and give
> It doesn't matter how you die but only how you live

A sense of frenzy builds out of the play's grotesque images of death. The obsession with killing evolves out of the climate of suffocation. "Men are most apt to kill or wish to kill when they feel themselves symbolically dying—that is, overcome by images of stasis, meaninglessness, and the separation from the larger currents of human life." [2] Even the snake—an escaped Air Force computer invented to trace UFOs—is struggling for its survival. The military has created the snake out of a desire to extend human power to control of the universe. The Air Force wants the snake back because it represents billions of research dollars; the snake's inventor, Dr. Vector, wants it back in order to justify his life's work and to calibrate the superhuman capabilities of his invention. As he explains to the Air Force officers:

> DR. VECTOR: At this stage it becomes apparent to me that all man-made efforts to produce this type of information were useless and that a much more sophisticated form of intelligence was necessary. A form of intelligence which, being triggered from the mind, would eventually, if allowed to exist on its own, transcend the barriers of human thought and penetrate an extraterrestrial consciousness.

The oppressiveness of the society's technology—the

death-oriented investment in military research and the military itself—becomes so large a threat that the radical despair turns from revolutionary plans to petty rebellions. The Young Man is a pawn for three black militants. Shepard introduces the audience to the trio as they discuss their plan at a desert hot-dog stand. Their political scheme is as pathetic and futile as the Weathermen's, but, like the Young Man, they have lost a sense of their identity in America and they are trying to forge a new one. Revolution gives their lives an immediate focus and destiny. The militants are very conspicuous guerrillas. Dressed in paramilitary fashion, they exist above ground in a daydream of underground activity. The carhop immediately assumes they are Panthers. They want lunch; she wants a soul talk. She too is looking for a sense of power and purpose. She imitates their rhetoric of revolt and imagines a revolutionary unity in a society which, like the snake, has been dramatically divided.

> CARHOP: Like I can really dig this whole unity thing that you guys are into but it seems like we could be doing something to help bind it all together. You know, I mean you people have such a groovy thing going. . . . We're not going to turn on any of these zombies. We gotta find our own people and turn ourselves on. Make something happen for us.

Her hyperbole is hilarious. In her eyes, the blacks as victims are the only hope of America's spiritual salvation. She sees only the relationship between purity and powerlessness. But when the blacks talk about their plans, the audience sees how deeply the society's oppression has affected them. One crazy scheme is topped by another:

DUDE: The pilots get a good taste of supersonic water. They start feeling funny. They hear voices. They see things in the air. They hear music. They get stoned like they never been before in their lives. . . . In the middle of the night they all get up in unison like Dracula and his sisters and walk straight into the night. They climb into their sleek F111s just south of Miami whereupon they land and await further instructions. . . .

BLADE: I don't know, it's like James Bond or something. Why don't we go in and take the thing over?

The blacks' scheme may seem outrageous, but the despair beneath it parallels the Yippie tactics in Chicago:

The list of Yippie projects, by no means exhaustive, included ten thousand nude bodies floating in protest in Lake Michigan; the mobilization of Yippie "hookers" to seduce delegates and slip LSD into their drinks; a squad of 230 "hyperpotent" hippie males assigned to the task of seducing the wives and daughters of delegates . . . the insertion of LSD into the city's water supply. . . . An emergency guard [of Chicago Police] was placed on the city's LSD-threatened water supply, just in case.[3]

The gestures become more preposterous as the society becomes more repressive. The victims become victimizers. In *Operation Sidewinder*, the ghoulish paradox in the Air Force plot is that there is a lack of humanity in the rebellion. In the name of life, the revolutionaries will take lives. The "heroism" of the radicals is not in their plan for society, but in taking *any* action at all. As the targets get larger, the possibilities for success get smaller. The desperation in the recent bombings that have terrified the nation comes out of the kind of manic anguish Shepard dramatizes. In both the stage and the real world, we witness the panic-stricken attempts of the drowning to find air, to rid themselves of society's death imprint. A terrorist letter (*The New York Times,* March 13, 1970) contains the pain, the dislocation, the mad disproportion Shepard evokes through the Young Man and the militant "cadre":

> This way of "life" is a way of death. To work for the industries of death is to murder. To know the torments Amerika inflicts on the Third World, but not to sympathize and identify, is to deny our right to love—to deny our own humanity. We refuse. In death-directed Amerika there is only one way to a life of love and freedom; to attack and destroy the forces of death and exploitation and to build a just society—revolution.
>
> —*(Signed)* REVOLUTIONARY FORCE 9

Shepard's Young Man, zonked on drugs and obsessed with his scheme, has tried and failed to find a place for himself in America. He sees his predicament clearly, but he cannot put a stop to historical momentum. Sitting with Honey in the desert, he says, "I am depressed, deranged, dehumanized, and damned." His anxiety comes from feeling the innocence and purity ripped from him by the society that betrays even the dreams it foists on its citizens in order to control them. Honey confesses that she and her husband were on their way to get a divorce. She is bored. She can't understand her aimlessness. But as she talks, Honey shows her sense of abandonment by describing dreams of largesse, safety, and hope which have fed the nation's mythology:

> HONEY: My mama said that sometimes . . . someday I'd make my living from my hair. . . . That I should come to Hollywood and the very next day, just from walking

around the streets and everything, that someone would see my hair and ask me to come and get a screen test. And that before very long I'd be famous and rich and everything.

For Honey and the Young Man, the only experience of America is loss. The play's episodic structure is a dreamlike correlative to the Young Man's sense of America. As one of the songs emphasizes, there is nothing in America to latch on to:

> I came here with my guidebook
> With my license in hand
> But the landing field keeps slipping out of line
> And this ain't what they told me I'd find
> The biggest laugh around here
> Is the changing ground here. . . .

When Honey asks the Young Man his name and his origins, he starts to freak out. He is everyman and no man; he is everywhere and nowhere:

YOUNG MAN: I am from the planet Krypton. No, I am from the Hollywood Hills. No. I am from Freak City. That's where I was raised anyway. . . . I am an American though. Despite what they say. In spite of the scandal. I am truly an American, I was made in America. Born, bred, and raised. I have American scars on my brain. Red, white, and blue. I bleed American blood. I dream American dreams. I fuck American girls. I devour the planet. I'm an earth eater.

The Young Man wants to swallow the world, to hold it within himself. He cannot relate to a life force within Amer-

ica. Like the rest of the people in Shepard's play, he belongs
to a country of aliens. A song crystallizes the Young Man's
predicament:

> I couldn't go back where I came from
> 'Cause that would just bring me back here
> And this is the place I was born, bred, and raised
> And it doesn't seem like I was ever here. . . .

The Young Man has witnessed the violence of the government toward peaceful protest. He is haunted by images
of political deception and emotional castration:

YOUNG MAN: The election oppression: Nixon, Wallace,
Humphrey. The headline oppression every morning with
one of their names on it. . . . And I was all set to watch
"Mission: Impossible" when Humphrey's flabby face
shows up for another hour's alienation session. Oh, please
say something different, something real, something—so
we can believe again. His squirmy little voice answers me,
"You can't always have everything your own way." And
the oppression of my fellow students becoming depressed.
Depressed. Despaired. Running out of gas. "We're not
going to win. There's nothing we can do to win." This is
how it begins, I see. We become so depressed we don't
fight any more. We're only losing a little, we say. It could
be so much worse. The soldiers are dying, the blacks are
dying, the children are dying. It could be so much worse.

Those bludgeoned and jailed for legally protesting the
1968 Chicago Democratic Convention are the Young
Man's ghosts. The government reacts with equal capri-
ciousness to legal or illegal protest. The Young Man's actions are an attempt to deny the lies of government, to mo-

bilize himself with an energy and force he cannot find in
the society. He feels invisible; the plot is a means of making
his presence felt.

But the Young Man's plan does not work. Mickey Free
does not make the drop. Instead, he takes the head of the
snake to the Spider Lady, the shaman of the Hopis. She immediately accepts this as an omen of their race's transcendence, the final struggle between the material and the spiritual world:

> SPIDER LADY: Once the two halves were joined, the people
> would be swept from the earth by a star, for they were to
> be saved from the destruction at hand. That soon after,
> the spirit snake would again be pulled in half by the evil
> ones and the Fourth World would come to an end. . . .

Mickey Free gives up guns and drugs, and awaits his spiritual transformation. Meanwhile, the blacks have sent the
Young Man and Honey back into the desert looking for the
sidewinder computer, which the blacks want for political
leverage. To the military, the snake is property; to the Young
Man and Honey, it is a way of getting themselves out of a
threatening jam; to Mickey Free, it is a hope of rebirth.

The CIA is brought into the case. Captain Bovine questions the prospector about the identity of the Young Man.
Behind Bovine's search for scapegoats is an insistence on
national purity, a dream he will not admit has been destroyed. His conspiratorial view of history reflects his own
consciousness of the society's deterioration. The Young
Man and the other renegades in Shepard's play use sex,
revolution, and drugs to get outside their flesh, to imitate
the longed-for rebirth. Captain Bovine faces the same prob-

lem, but has a different solution. He is also confused about the present, but he wants to return to a past he imagines was secure:

> CAPTAIN BOVINE: Over the past few years there's been a general breakdown of law and order and a complete disrespect for the things we hold sacred since our ancestors founded this country. This country needs you, Billy. It needs your help to help root out these subversive, underground creeps and wipe the slate clean once and for all. . . . Things have stayed the same for too long. It's time for a change.

Captain Bovine is talking the language of annihilation. Shepard etches the contours of what is emerging in America: a society more afraid of its dissenters than its corruption. Bovine wants a pure society, a nation as pristine as it was when the first settlers came here. Yet he cannot see how far that society has strayed from its original dreams. Richard Harris reports in his book *Justice* that Attorney General Richard G. Kleindienst had "reportedly promised to crack down on 'draft dodgers,' on 'anarchistic kids,' and on 'militants' of all persuasions, and this threat led some high members of the Justice Department to wonder if all dissent was to be stifled on the pretext that it amounted to subversion." [4] Harris quotes from a report in the *Chicago Daily News*:

> Undercover police investigations in Illinois are at an all-time high. In the Chicago area alone, more than 1000 men from the FBI and various other federal, state, county, and city agencies are working on supersecret assignments. "Our growing concern about subversives and militants with their talk of armed revolution has brought us a temporary shift

away from organized crime," said Illinois State Police Supt.
James T. McGuire. "I've never seen anything like the intensity of the current investigations in all my years in law en-
forcement. . . ." [5]

Operation Sidewinder dramatizes the yearning for a new history and the search for new symbols to inhabit the world.
Like the Young Man, Shepard is fascinated by Indian culture. The apocalyptic vision prophesied by the Spider Lady
is acted out on stage—a fantasy enactment of our cosmic
longings and fears, as in a science-fiction thriller. This theatrical tactic reflects Shepard's own desire to have symbols
transformed from death-giving to life-giving. The sidewinder begins the play as an evil omen associated with a
Christian tradition which has linked the snake with death,
and ends as a symbol of rebirth. At first, Honey and the
Young Man do not react like Mickey Free when they bring
the body of the snake back into the Hopi camp:

MICKEY: You are the Pahana! You have come! You have
brought us our salvation!
YOUNG MAN: Wait a minute! Wait a minute! That's mine!
That belongs to somebody else! Mickey! Cut it out! You
can't have that snake . . . That's a machine, you creep!
It's not real. The Air Force cooked it up to trace flying
saucers! The spades want to trace the Air Force. I want it
because it means my life if I don't get it back to them.

The Hopi snake dance begins, with the sidewinder incorporated into the ritual. Shepard is interweaving cultures:
that of the Indian, with his sense of sacredness in life, with
that of a modern society which has lost that reverence. The
play's final image brings the outlandish plot to a brilliant
epiphany: the world of spirit (the Indians) challenged by

the material world (the military). Paratroopers, claiming the sidewinder as their property, interrupt the snake dance just as the snake's head is being reunited with its body, fulfilling the Hopi prophecy of transcendence. Honey and the Young Man have now allied themselves with the Indians, discovering an identity and a sense of spiritual continuity. The radical scheme and the drugs are abandoned for a mystical "grace." To the Indians, Honey and the Young Man are saviors; but they are also saved. Chanting, while the soldiers fire into the crowd, the Indians cling to the snake. No one falls. Finally, a soldier wrestles the snake away. He rips off its head. His victory is the destruction of the world. The Indians, untouched, move toward their salvation; the soldiers twitch in a violent death. Smoke fills the theater. The final poetic image anticipates the apocalypse and friezes the true believer.

American theater is threatened by the same *rigor mortis* as the society. For both to survive, a new flexibility must evolve. To achieve this, the playwright and his audience must take risks. Not all theatrical probings will be successful, and those that succeed may be flawed as literature. But the theater needs distinct, ruthless visions like those of Shepard and Feiffer to shock its audiences from their life-sleep, that numbing complacency by which they survive the nation's spiritual decay by pretending it doesn't exist.

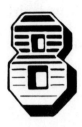

Neil Simon
and Woody Allen:
Images of Impotence

"Make voyages. Attempt them. There is nothing else." The words are Lord Byron's in Tennessee Williams' *Camino Real*, which in 1953 closed quickly on Broadway, where imaginative voyages, even then, were rare. There is a heroic sentiment in the lines, a youthful faith in human resilience and courage which should be the emblem of American theater. Yet Broadway snuffs out those plays which are the most playful—those which challenge the world to see itself afresh. The list of high-quality casualties on Broadway is long: S. J. Perelman's *The Beauty Part* (1963), Jules Feiffer's *Little Murders* (1967), John Guare's *Cop-Out* (1969), Arthur Kopit's *Indians* (1970), Michael Weller's *Moonchildren* (1972). What survives on Broadway are plays about its audience: the comedies of Neil Simon (*Last of the Red Hot Lovers*, *Plaza Suite*, and *Promises, Promises*) and Woody Allen's

Play It Again, Sam. These long-run Broadway successes offer up—in laughter—images of impotence. The plays are victims of their subject matter: the sense of life on stage shrinks as the characters shrink from life. Questionable as they might be as art, the plays cannot be discounted as social documents. This is the theater of the silent majority. In the humor are a moral confusion and spiritual dread which show the foundations of the reactionary wilderness that America is becoming, and the unthinking violence which is condoned as normalcy.

Stage comedy has ossified with the society. The earlier comedians—Bert Lahr, Bobby Clark, the Marx Brothers—dealt (as in the present comic situations) with failure. They had a frantic and anarchic energy. They mangled language. They brushed up against the world. In the pratfall and the malaprop, there was humiliation, but in rebounding there was a joyous implication of power and hope. The humor was child's play, interested in discovery and challenge. Although the characters they portrayed were often inept and daydreamy, the comedians gave them a certain nobility. They offered an image of comic control. Their entire performing mechanism (face, voice, body) implied a vision of the world.

The early comedians were young, inquisitive survivors. In the contemporary Broadway comedies, none of their curiosity or resilience remains. Movement is minimal; the actors seem not to exist from the neck down. Whereas the earlier comedians were "personalities," Neil Simon and Woody Allen offer images of people who have no "identity" and no means of controlling experience. They have no unity with their bodies. Although most of them lust for sex and new experiences, they are firmly wedded to the bourgeois life. They are not outsiders like the early clowns. They are powerless to change, or at least they have convinced themselves that they are. The situation obsesses Neil Simon, whose plays report what he sees in America's middle-class way of life.

> I'm terribly conscious of the powerlessness of the people in the plays. But this is basic structural dramatic writing. Character is fate. People have to be destroyed by their own characters; they must not be able to cope with it. Almost every character in my plays knows exactly what his problem is. It's not the case of not knowing who they are. In *The Odd Couple*, Oscar says to Felix, "You mean you have no idea of changing." And Felix says, "I am what I am." He knows exactly who he is and cannot change it. When I look around in life, most people who are in trouble know what the problems are. They say, "There's nothing I can do about it. That's the way I am." This becomes sadder to people over forty because they feel their characters are determined . . . they're trapped. The trap is themselves, not necessarily life.*

But both Simon and his characters forget that man is evolved by society. Deprived of a strong sense of themselves, Simon's characters are fighting to stand still. They don't want change because, uncertain of who they are, they are more frightened of what they might become. In the ailing world of these comedies, experience has been quarantined. The characters have no sense of destiny in the world or continuity in history. In a nation where, in 1968, 57 per cent of the electorate voted for either Richard Nixon or George Wallace, Simon's stage separation of character from society chronicles the reactionary impulse which disguises impotence with pragmatism. The plays see a predicament, but,

*All Neil Simon quotations are from a conversation with the author.

like the characters in them, are not willing to probe the sources or consequences of despair. Simon is conscious of his artistic limitations.

> I think the society is the result of what my particular character is, magnified many times. When you have to deal with life in general—the society—I can't deal with it. I have to get down to the specifics of character. The other thing out there does not interest me. Life in society, class revolution, generation—I leave it for those who are interested in it . . .

The impulse of the most successful Broadway comedy writer, then, is not to confront the world but to shore it up. Yet the comic situations betray a sickness which goes beyond human foibles to social madness.

I

The characters in Broadway comedies are the *castrati* of capitalism. There is no heroic possibility in their work. Bureaucracy splits up manpower, pools human resources. These Broadway comic stereotypes' tasks are small, their alienation compounded by their reverence for the bourgeois credo: efficiency, stamina, compliance, and safety. Yet this leaves them strangely dissatisfied. Life is experienced as separation from the environment and from the body. They feel small and weak. In *Promises, Promises* (a musical based on Billy Wilder and I. A. L. Diamond's screenplay for *The Apartment*), the hero—Chuck—lends the keys to his apartment to company executives. He wants to get ahead; they want to get laid. The frantic sexual merry-go-round is an indication of an impotence in corporate life. Chuck, of course, will never realize this, and his experience of the world epitomizes this debility:

CHUCK: The main problem with working as a hundred-and-
twelve-dollar-a-week accountant in a seventy-two-story
insurance company with assets of over three billion dollars that employs thirty-one thousand two hundred and
fifty-two people . . . is that it makes a person feel so God-
awful puny. . . .

If you've noticed I'm the kind of person that people
don't notice. I wish I were sitting out there with you so I
could take a look at me and figure out what went wrong.

A Lilliputian in the Land of Plenty, Chuck cannot im-
press himself on others. In *Last of the Red Hot Lovers*, Barney
Cashman, a forty-seven-year-old restaurateur who decides
to have an affair, observes, "Life has not been particularly
kind to me, in fact, it goes out of its way to ignore me." The
line gets applause. Cashman is faceless and he is frantically
trying to break into the world. Woody Allen's surrogate,
Allan Felix, in *Play It Again, Sam* is a pill-popping neurotic,
petrified of the world and fearful of his incapacity to deal
with it. ("I'm a disgrace to my sex. I should work in an Ara-
bian palace as a eunuch.") Felix lives in his fantasies to escape the limp facts of his existence. His ex-wife haunts his
dreams and incites his secondhand life: "You like movies
because you're one of life's great watchers. I'm not like that.
I'm a doer. I want to participate."

But the comic characters on Broadway can't participate.
Vicarious experience becomes their real experience in a
world they cannot mold. They are trapped and confused,
hiding in their rooms and in their dreams. This schizophrenia is physicalized on stage. Their dreams are tangible: in
Play It Again, Sam, Allan Felix talks to and sees Humphrey
Bogart; Chuck in *Promises, Promises* makes up imaginary
conversations with a girl he admires and hears her speak

back to him; in *Last of the Red Hot Lovers*, Barney Cashman's liaisons are a restaging of his "fantasies, secret dreams, experiencing things, emotions, stimulants . . . [he's] never experienced before." In the laughter, there is a hollow despair. Barney Cashman senses part of the predicament —fantasy is never sufficient: "So many things I wanted to do . . . but I'll never do 'em . . . So many places I wanted to see . . . I'll never see 'em. . . . Trapped. . . . We're all trapped. . . . Help! Help!" Groping to recover his diminishing humanity, Cashman invests himself with potency and significance. He wants to seduce his best friend's wife, Jeanette. She balks and asks him what's the matter:

> BARNEY: Nothing's the matter with me, sweetheart. I'm with it! I'm now! I'm here where it's happening. Jeanette, where the hell are you? Now are you going to take off that dress or do I rip it off with my fingers?

The less certain Barney is of his position in the world and of his emotional and moral roots, the more frantic and violent he becomes. The characters in the Broadway comedies are numb to themselves, blunted by their values as well as their work.

II

The dread of life attaches itself to the body.
—KARL JASPERS, *Man in the Modern Age*

Broadway comedies are preoccupied with sex, but the characters dread their flesh because they dread themselves.

They have no real physical focus. Sensation is a memory. Barney Cashman probes the needs of his first seducee, Elaine Navazio:

ELAINE: I get cravings.
BARNEY: You mean, to eat?
ELAINE: To eat, to touch, to smell, to see, to do. . . . A sensual, physical pleasure that can only be satisfied at that moment.
BARNEY: You mean like after a game of handball, a cold Pepsi?

Cashman's body is as crustaceous as his response. He has no control over his body or his life. In *Play It Again, Sam*, Allan Felix is not even sure he still has a penis:

ALLAN: Now what?
BOGART: Tell her that she moves something in you that you can't control.
ALLAN: You're kidding?

Allan recognizes only negative qualities in his body. At one point he is so sexually confused that he says to a fantasy female figure, "I love you Miss Whoever-You-Are. I want to have your baby."

Sex is a means of suspending time and finding a union with the world. But the flesh is a reminder of the pressure of time and man's decay. Cashman continually sniffs his fingers for a fish smell which would offend his lover; Felix is petrified of the death and ugliness of his body. He wants to cover it with deodorant.

BOGART: For christ sake, you're going to smell like a French cathouse.
ALLAN: I need them.

BOGART: Why? You ashamed to sweat? . . . Y'know, kid, somewhere in life you got turned around.

ALLAN: . . . He's right. A lot of girls get turned on by a masculine earthy quality. I shouldn't have put so much Binaca under my arms. I want to create a good subliminal impression.

In *Plaza Suite*'s first play, "A Visitor from Mamaroneck," Karen wants to make her husband, Sam, recall the playful early days of their marriage. At fifty-one he is fighting old age, working hard to keep in shape, longing for the energy and the chance "to do it all over again." The humiliation of the flesh is in its loss of resilience:

KAREN: I like you flabby.

SAM: What does that mean?

KAREN: It means I like you flabby. I admit you look like one of the Pepsi generation, but it seems unnatural to me. A man of your age ought to have a couple of pounds of skin hanging over his belt.

SAM: Well, I'm sorry to disappoint you.

KAREN: I'm not disappointed. I'm uncomfortable. I watch you when you get undressed at night. Nothing moves. You're vacuum packed. When you open your belt I expect it to go like a can of coffee—Pzzzzz.

The comic characters are literally and figuratively rootless. For coherent ties with the world, they substitute moments of passion. They want to connect but they are shackled by values that prevent fulfillment. Even when the characters are sexually successful, there is an ambiguity about their victory. Chuck wins "the girl of his dreams" without ever having touched her. Allan Felix has an affair with his friend's wife, Linda. She claims he's fantastic in bed, but in the longed-for union, he wasn't even thinking of her:

> LINDA: What were you thinking of while we were doing it?
> ALLAN: Willie Mays. . . .
> LINDA: You always think of baseball players when you're making love?
> ALLAN: It keeps me going.
> LINDA: I couldn't figure out why you kept yelling "Slide."

Unlike Willie Mays, Allan is no long hitter. But his response mirrors how much the act of intercourse is intended to bring him back to a sense of his power and his history. As Alan Harrington has written:

> The sexual partner turns into a stand-in for various dream figures, phantasms in a stage-managed resurrection. These figures—father, mother, brute, victim, amazon, master, slave, child, disciple—are all agents of immortality to be conquered or succumbed to many times over in order that the pilgrim without faith may symbolically die and live again. In consequence, the lover whose once-immortal soul is gone does not so much possess his companion as his own dreams. The loved one's role becomes less that of being loved than one of assisting the other's desire to live on—a sort of sexual travel agent helping to arrange divine trips.[1]

In *Last of the Red Hot Lovers*, the spectacle of impotence is taken to its extreme. From the beginning of his search for illicit sex Cashman has feared the worst.

> BARNEY: . . . Would you be a lot happier if I started ripping off your clothes and jumping all over you? No hello, no nothing. Just the pure, physical animal act. Is that what you prefer?
> ELAINE: Well, it would be a way of breaking the ice.

BARNEY: Because, if that's what you want I certainly could accommodate you. I mean there's no problem in that area, is there?

But Barney cannot get laid. In desperation, he calls his wife and asks her to meet him at his sequestered apartment. The woman whom he has described as "not extraordinary, not what you would call an exciting, vivacious woman, but one who is kind, considerate, devoted and that I happen to love," becomes in that gesture a mere acquaintance. By pretending that this is an illicit liaison, Cashman illustrates his profound confusion. In a love relationship, the man becomes aware of himself through his partner. Since Cashman does not know who he is, genuine love is a threat. Cashman's search for sex is really a search for himself. But even Cashman's wife won't come to the apartment. Neil Simon sees the moment as one of total psychic disaster.

> He has nothing left, not even a dream. This guy's wiped out. He's not going home and saying, "I'm going to live a happy life and I'm going to be a happy man from now on." He's faced a certain truth and now he's going to have to deal only in truth and no more in dream. And so it's going to get worse for him. He'll have to cope with it. He's not going to pieces, and he's not going to kill himself. He'll have to come to grips with it somehow. Maybe he'll manufacture another type of dream. Maybe he'll say, "I'll become a big business-man."

But there are contradictions in Simon's statement. Work and dream are sexual surrogates. "Truth" cannot be faced except as fantasy. Simon, who sees his characters as funny-sad, does not admit the depth of their sickness. Yet there is nothing sane in their allegiance to bourgeois values. R. D. Laing has pointed this out:

The "normal" state of affairs is to be so immersed in one's immersion in social phantasy systems that one takes them to be real. Many images have been used to remind us of this condition. We are dead, but think we are alive. We are asleep, but think we are awake. We are dreaming, but take our dream to be reality. We are the halt, the lame, blind, deaf, the sick. But we are doubly unconscious. We are so ill that we no longer feel ill, as in many terminal illnesses. We are mad but have no insight.[2]

This is an accurate diagnosis of the characters in the Broadway comedies.

III

The language of these comic figures is as restricted and banal as they are. There is little wit or irony. In a world aspiring to moderation, language loses its sense of life and its cogency. Both Chuck in *Promises, Promises* and Allan in *Play It Again, Sam* are so nervous about what to say that they hold conversations with themselves. Their words do not touch the world outside and they admit it. Sensuous language is used in mock-poetic terms, an exercise in salesmanship, not discovery. Barney Cashman composes menus for his restaurant: "I don't write visual. I write for the ear. 'Sweet succulent savory swordfish steak.' " His ear is dead, and so is his language. Although words pour out of Cashman, they become disguises rather than revelations. Language is to be feared rather than relished. Elaine, the ferocious sexual athlete, has no time for Cashman's fastidiousness:

> ELAINE: I bet I could say three words right now that would turn your blue suit into a Glen Plaid. . . . I'm gonna say

it. I'm going to say a word now. You want to put your
hands over your ears?
BARNEY: Hey, come on, Elaine, I don't think this is
funny. . . .
ELAINE: I'm saying it. . . . Screw!
BARNEY *(double take)*: Asshole! I can do it too. . . .

This paltry verbal surprise indicates Cashman's impotence. The words offend because they imply a failure. One
way to forget personal limitations is to control the ways of
talking about them. This same mentality is extended to our
political structure. At a time when the nation has lost its
sense of destiny, believing in its goodness but committed to
increasing social atrocities, President Nixon asks Americans
to swallow their indignation:

> In these difficult years, America has suffered from a fever of
> words; from inflated rhetoric that promises more than it can
> deliver; from angry rhetoric that fans discontent into ha-
> tred; from bombastic rhetoric that postures instead of per-
> suading: We cannot learn from one another until we stop
> shouting at each other—until we speak quietly enough so
> that our words can be heard as well as our voices.[3]

At a lower timbre, language loses its threat; political betrayal and public brutality seem less ominous. Under the
banner of normalcy, society, like Broadway's stage characters, hides a deeper sickness from itself. When Spiro Agnew
criticized television's image of America, he eliminated the
sense of failure, but not the cause:

> Normality has become the nemesis of the network news.
> Now the upshot of all this controversy is that a narrow and
> distorted picture of America often emerges from the tele-
> vised news. . . .

> —*The New York Times*, November 14, 1969

The political circus, like the Broadway comedies, is cor-
seted into a deadly decorum.

In "Visitor from Forest Hills" (*Plaza Suite*), the father of
the bride-to-be urges his daughter out of a bathroom, where
she has locked herself before the wedding. Nothing works.
Finally he calls the bridegroom. The diminutive young man
walks in and goes to the door: "Mimsey? . . . This is Bor-
den. . . . Cool it!" He walks out. Seconds later the daughter opens the door, radiant and ready to be married. The
father is dumbfounded. "I break every bone and you come
out for 'Cool it?' . . . That's how he communicates? That's
the brilliant understanding between two people?"

But the father's understanding of his wife, Norma, and
family is no more sensitive. Language becomes a series of
demands and silences. The wife chronicles the brutality:

> NORMA: . . . All right, so we yell and scream a little. So we
> fight and curse and aggravate each other. So you blame
> me for being a lousy mother and I accuse you of being a
> rotten husband. It doesn't mean we're not happy. . . .
> Does it? . . . Well? . . . Does it?

IV

In the Broadway comedies, the characters are enslaved
by the benefits of the American way of life. Tired, belea-
guered, confused, they acquiesce to whatever happens to
them, never pushing a serious question to the point where
they might discover an answer. The fiancée who barri-
cades herself in the bathroom in "Visitor from Forest Hills"
because "she's afraid of what they're going to become," is
finally coaxed into a tepid marriage with a boy as inept and

frigid as her father. The daughter's recalcitrance is the only moment of protest in the comedies. In "Visitor from Mamaroneck" (*Plaza Suite*) the wife is perplexed by the unhappiness of her marriage. She has equated acquisitions with spiritual liberation:

> KAREN: What's wrong? We have a twelve-room house in the country, two sweet children, a maid who doesn't drink. Is there something missing?
> SAM: I—don't know.

Karen accepts sadness as well as injustice. Her husband is too busy with his work to enjoy their twenty-third wedding anniversary. Sex and companionship are memories. He screams at her to be quiet. "I'll even take the nastiness," she says. "It's not too much, but it's a start." The loneliness behind her words may not be profound but it is pertinent. Without a focus to her life or a sense of her own potential, she feels utterly useless. Her husband confesses he has been sleeping with his secretary:

> SAM: What are we going to do?
> KAREN: Well, you're taken care of. You're having an affair. I'm the one who needs an activity.

The joke brings down the house. Karen's surrender to emotional emasculation disguises weakness as "niceness." In *Promises, Promises*, Chuck (the quintessential good guy) is stood-up, double-crossed, and confounded by the girl he loves. He is prepared to give her up and let his Lothario boss marry her rather than tip the corporate boat. In the end, she comes to Chuck. The moral is clear; weakness brings its own reward. Allan Felix (*Play It Again, Sam*) discovers that he can succeed with his failure. He casts off his daydreams of Bogart, saying, "The secret's not being you, it's being me. True, you're not too tall and kinda ugly. But I'm short enough and ugly enough to succeed myself." The next moment the doorbell rings and a gorgeous girl walks in, brushing him with her body. A happy ending, but his impotence is disguised, not dealt with.

The characters do not fight back or take charge of their lives. They are richer but still forgotten Americans, easily manipulated because they are prepared to accept anything which will give them a sense of direction in the world. Their boredom reflects their spiritual floundering. Jeanette confides a special American middle-class despair to Barney in *Last of the Red Hot Lovers*:

> It's waking up each morning of your life not wanting anything, not hoping, not caring, not needing. You don't pray for happiness because you don't believe it exists and you don't wish for death because if you don't exist then death is meaningless. All that is left is a quiet, endless, bottomless, relentless, eternal infinite gloom. . . .

This speech may exaggerate melancholy for laughs, but it implies the lack of freedom in a life that does not see struggle as an essential ingredient of self-fulfillment. The predicament of America's white middle class is depicted in the comedies. There is quarreling but no quest. The characters, like the audiences the plays are about, have traded liberty for comfort. Karl Jaspers has written: "The essence of freedom is struggle: it does not want to appease but to intensify the contest, does not want to acquiesce but to enforce open demonstrations." [4]

By being true to the bondage of his characters, Neil

Simon acknowledges their impotence, but is forced into a theatrical style which, in offering genuine insight into the shallows of society, is also a slavery to them:

> There will be a point in the writing of a play when I say to myself: "Well, maybe the character should fight his situation." And he says: "OK, I'm going to break away from this." And I start to play around with this, to oppose it exactly as you say. But it's not truthful. It just wouldn't happen. Let's say Barney Cashman says: "To hell with my job at the seafood restaurant—I'm going to break away." That's a very theatrical idea but it's not a very truthful one. It's not the way life would go; it's away from truth, and I'm trying to write the truth as it applies to that segment of the world.

V

Broadway comedies seem to be apolitical, but they are not. They habituate audiences to patterns of avoidance that feed a profound social violence. Philip Slater writes:

> If America gained the energetic and the daring we also . . . gained a critically undue proportion of persons who, when faced with a difficult situation, tended to chuck the whole thing and flee to a new environment. Escaping, evading, and avoiding are responses which lie at the base of much that is peculiarly American—the suburb, the automobile, the self-service store, and so on.[5]

On stage, the audience can applaud the superficiality they have helped to create and call its evocation "entertainment." Broadway comedies are symptomatic of America's frantic pursuit of happiness which demands a pathological unawareness of social failure in order to feel good about itself. Devoid of satire and sting, the comedies sweep aside moral problems and social observation in the same spirit that the blacks and Indians have been ghettoized: out of sight, out of mind. There is no rejuvenation through the Broadway comic experience, only sedation. The impotence which on stage is excused by laughter turns, in society, to political madness. Evasion becomes a way of life. Traumatic failures of the democratic ideal are blocked from public consciousness and dreams displace cruel fact—the Gulf of Tonkin, the My Lai massacre. History becomes a scenario rewritten to justify the impotence of leadership: Julius Hoffman's Chicago court, Spiro Agnew's broadsides to the media, the Harrisburg conspiracy trial. The only way to deny failure is to avoid the facts of life.

Broadway comedy, like its audience, is fulfilling a death wish, a sad, perhaps prophetic, omen of the society as well as the stage.

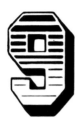

Mystery on Stage

Don't they know how bad we need men of
. . . mystery, honorable mystery, persons of
the proper secret, and not those with it wished
or pushed upon them. . . .

—JOHN FORD NOONAN, *The Year Boston Won the Pennant*

"If it is true that the ability to be puzzled is the beginning of wisdom," wrote Erich Fromm, "then this is a sad commentary on the wisdom of modern man. Whatever the merits of our high degree of literacy and universal education, we have lost the gift of being puzzled." [1] Unconsciously, theater has attempted to demystify the human situation, the language, and even the body. (*Oh! Calcutta!* offers sex without pursuit, flesh without mystery; *The Great White Hope* and *All Over*, typical of more "serious" stage literature, offer characters who explain their motivation like salesmen for the self.) Yet the theater's greatest potential for laughter and terror evolves from the secret statement of personality and the mercurial fabric of experience. There is an enigmatic quality to life which the conventions of stage exposition, plot, and focus often deny. Harold Pinter has explained the philosophical framework behind mystery on stage and its unsettling threat to any modern audience:

> Who are we to say the one thing is the consequence of another? . . . What reason have we to suppose that life is so neat and tidy? The most we know for sure is that the things which have happened have happened in a certain order; any connections we think we see, or choose to make, are pure guesswork. Life is much more mysterious than plays make it out to be. And it is this mystery which fascinates me: what happens between words, what happens when no words are spoken.[2]

Middle-class entertainment, like bourgeois life, aspires to a security and unreflective contentment with the world. Most theater reflects this static demand for the illusion of coherence. By avoiding mystery, theater avoids seriousness. In resolving all conflicts, theater abdicates the painful weight of dream. Artaud's accusation is still true: "Theater has lost the feeling for seriousness on one hand and for laughter on the other; because it has broken away from gravity, from effects that are immediate and painful—in a word, from Danger." [3]

To put mystery back into language and gesture is to renew their potency. This has been a goal of the best avant-garde theater. Deprived of familiar signposts, the imagination is forced more vigorously into play. Joe Chaikin, director of the Open Theatre, has said:

> I'd like to see each play have its own code in the use of words. Each play is only involved in its special poetry. It would become a kind of language, with the syntax carrying

a special kind of meaning. The words have special meaning to the audience and the actor. That's what the playwright, finally, has to do. I despair of conversation and conventional language. It just doesn't carry meaning any more. It's facile.[4]

A secret language "implies the abolition of time—of history concentrated in language." [5] In the Open Theatre's *Terminal*, a theater piece exploring the idea of death, an Executed Man speaks and a woman gripping an upright bed counterpoints his speech with nonsense words. Her song evokes a profound longing:

> My prison's made of steel;
> yours is in your head. . . .

The sound of the wooden bed rocking against the floor grows louder.

The song fills the woman; it uses her voice to sing itself.

The words of the song are repeated over and over again with various intentions.

The meaning of the words is secondary to the range of human emotions which can be expressed through them.

> A-nee Ma-a-meen
> A-nee Ma-a-meen
> A-nee Ma-a-meen
> A-nee Ma-a-meen, etc.

The image is presented as symbol and statement. "In a symbol there is concealment and yet revelation; hence, therefore, by silence and speech acting together, comes a double significance." [6] The actors in this kind of theater must find sources of articulation which are extraordinary; so too must the audience. "What we know of another person comes through the voice and the body," says Chaikin in his book *The Presence of the Actor*. "If the voice of the actor is limited and the body is fastened to the repertoire of sitting, standing and fending off, there is the same potential for articulation as there is over coffee and a danish."

Performance theater emphasizes the silent language of the body. And many new playwrights in America have begun to take theatrical experience into the realm of the irrational. Sam Shepard, Robert Coover, John Ford Noonan create mysteries which often confound critics but release a profound source of energy and ideas for the artist and audience.

I

Modern audiences value "make-believe," but rarely submit to it. When the curtain goes up on a realistic set and people on stage merely mirror the ideas and attitudes of our daily life, what is there for an audience to imagine? Mystery is a goad to imagination: it transforms theater into the purest and profound kind of play—hide-and-seek. Through mystery, the ritual function of theater is renewed. Unfettered from the mundane world of fact, the audiences can accept the inconceivable. They are open to the universe and to themselves. The unconscious is allowed to deploy its special knowledge without reference to the here and now, not couched in language of the intellect. And the stage, by allowing and structuring these moments of imaginative freedom, becomes a mode of the sacred.

Plays which embrace mystery acknowledge no absolute

or decisive knowledge, only private discoveries. There is more to cognition than what conscious thought provides. The subject of Pinter's plays is not only the mystery of human personality but the limitations of our modes of per̄ceiving it. We want to compartmentalize and define what is elusive and, because unknown, threatening. Pinter's orchestration of silences and pauses serves a larger end by dramatizing people making life-decisions on the spur of the moment. In these silences—where words are still reverberating with innuendo—each character recoups, realigns, reconsiders, and finally responds. No moment is ever certain and no object what it seems to be. As Ruth demonstrates to the admiring male household in *The Homecoming*, they must live with the ambiguity imagination forces on them:

> Look at me. I . . . move my leg. That's all it is. But I wear . . . underwear . . . which moves with me . . . it . . . captures your attention. Perhaps you misinterpret. The action is simple. It's a leg . . . moving. My lips move. Why don't you restrict . . . your observations to that? Perhaps the fact they move is more significant . . . than the words which come through them. You must bear that . . . possibility . . . in mind.

To accept mystery is to affirm a process and not a result. Mystery on stage reflects a psychic truth which cannot be substantiated by science. This often makes the efficient theatergoer uncomfortable. His imagination at play has been warped by the systems which manipulate it at work. In a world dominated by technique, man has lost touch with primordial mystery.

> Technique worships nothing, respects nothing. It has a single role: to strip off externals, to bring everything to light,

and by rational use transform everything into means. More than science, which limits itself to explaining "how," technique *desacrilizes* because it demonstrates (by evidence and not by reason, through use and not through books) that mystery does not exist. Science brings to the light of day everything man had believed sacred.[7]

Science fiction is an attempt to unite the culture's passion for technique with its still deeper need for mystery. Sam Shepard's *Operation Sidewinder* juxtaposes the world of technology with the sacred, mystic universe of Hopi ritual. The play dramatizes the triumph of the sacred over technique. The play enters mythic terrain and yearns for a time that is "other than that of 'secular duration.' "[8] One rock song asks to banish time and its watchdog, memory.

> I used to walk on water too
> and float above the sand.
> And hang the stars like diamonds on my
> outstretched greedy hands.
> But I've forgotten how that game goes
> I disremember quite well.
>
> And did you ever do whatever thing
> it is you're for?
> Or does an old idea like that have meaning
> anymore?
> The maybe that I loved has gone, but where?
> I disremember quite well.

In *The Unseen Hand*, Shepard finds a theatrical situation which allows past, present, and future to coalesce. Here, the dead are awakened. Three nineteenth-century desperadoes

are called back to life to help Willie—a refugee from another planet—fight the oppression of the Silent Ones from
his native Nogoland. Willie is immortal; but he is punished
by "excruciating muscle spasms and nightmare visions" for
his imaginative powers. "Whenever our thoughts transcend
those of the magicians the Hand squeezes down and forces
our minds to contract into non-preoccupation." Neverthe-
less, Willie enacts many mythic patterns. He makes the old
drunk—Blue—young again. The stage directions dramatize
the mysteries of this rebirth:

> WILLIE *goes into another seizure but different this time. It's as though
> thousands of electric volts were being transmitted from* WILLIE *to*
> BLUE. *It should look like waves of shock being transformed. First*
> WILLIE *trembles, then* BLUE. BLUE *gradually becomes younger, until
> at the end he is a young man of about thirty.*

As the men plot to liberate Nogoland, they are inter-
rupted by the Kid, a Midwestern cheerleader who has run
away from the taunting pranks of an opposing team. His
language is stamped with the rhythms of rote learning and
an intractable materialism. He talks of the technique of
guerrilla warfare, but distrusts change. He lures the group
into accepting him, and then holds them at gunpoint.

> THE KID: Shut up! Shut up! I'll kill you all! I'll kill you.
> . . . This is my home. Don't make fun of my home. I was
> born and raised here . . . I love the foothills and the
> drive-in movies and the bowling alleys and the football
> games and the drag races and the girls and the donut
> shop and the High School and the Junior College and the
> Junior Chamber of Commerce and the Key Club and the
> Letterman's Club and the Kiwanis. . . .

The Kid's riff rambles on—a concrete word-picture of Midwestern life. Willie counteracts it and transforms the moment by speaking a magical language that terrifies the Kid and silences him.

> WILLIE: Asuza evol i. Dnatsrednu tnac uoy gnihtemos staht. Ti evol i. Ereh desiar dna nrob saw i. Emoh ym fo nuf ekam tnod . . .

Shepard intends this to be "a strange ancient language," which is an indication of Willie's return to the past. The fiction of a regression to a primitive tongue is a widespread pattern, shared by "a fairly large number of people ranging from the most primitive to the most civilized . . . [who] made use of solemn recitation of the cosmogonic myth as a therapeutic method." [9]

> WILLIE: . . . Emoh ym si siht. Uoy, llik lli. Lla uoy llik lli. Pu tuhs! Pu tuhs! Free! Free! Free!

Willie shouts his freedom. The Hand is in his control. His people in Nogoland are freed by the mystic power of his thought.

> It was all in my brain the whole time. In my mind. The ancient language of the Nogo. Right in my brain. I've destroyed them by breaking free of the Hand. They have no control. We can do what we want! We're free to do what we want!

On one level, Willie's statement is Shepard's message, but the form of the play goes still deeper. The key to spiritual freedom is in ourselves. We must embrace and respect the cosmic mysteries and work our way back to our emotional beginnings. The responsibility of the theater is to provide images which stimulate this spiritual journey.

II

A materialist culture longs to endow people with almost superhuman capacities of strength and wisdom. Once created, these cultural icons substitute for psychic fulfillment in an age of fragmentation. Modern man, seeking new sources of energy and creative power, constructs his heroes (Martin Luther King, John F. Kennedy, Malcolm X) only to destroy them, offended by an impossible purity and afraid of betrayal. Contemporary American theater's analysis of the communal need for and the creation of almost immortal figures and ideals acknowledges the debt of the unconscious in shaping man's inner landscape and also sets theater a higher task: to create "the invisible dimension, the not yet realized; leaving a space for the new." [10] To comment on legend, the stage must find forms of presentation which break down the literal and open play to the world of spirits and shadows that contain the religious underpinnings of legendary figures and legendary events.

In *The Kid*, a one-act play, Robert Coover explores the mysterious will to believe that produces heroes. His play dramatizes the process by which the profane is transformed into the sacred. He re-enacts the ritual duel between the Bad Man and the Sheriff. Coover offers an audience the externals of the old Western melodrama. His intention is not an easy parody of familiar forms; instead, he wants to expose the mysterious need behind them. The cowpokes in the saloon function as a chorus. They talk in simple sentences; no man is differentiated from another. There are also three

Belle Starrs, emphasizing the dream quality of the event.
The play begins with the exciting news that the Kid is coming to town. The Sheriff has sworn to gun him down. Yet
despite the Kid's outrageous "evil," the cattletown chorus
idealizes him. The Kid embodies and justifies their own values. His accomplishments give them energy and they try to
immortalize him in a song which is part of the process of
myth-making. Before the Kid arrives in town, the cowpokes
sing of their "saint's" grace and glory.

> He's kilt Apaches, Cayuses
> And Potawatami papooses
> And buggered the Chickasaw chiefs!
> Rid the country of snakes,
> And shit in the lakes,
> And hung all the schoolmarms and thiefs. . . .
>
> Jist blam! blam! blam!
> And he don't give a damn!
> He's the Savior of the West
>   He's the Savior of the West!

When he pushes through the saloon's swinging doors, the
Kid is radiant. Dressed in white, glistening in light, Coover's stage directions describe him as "a real impressive piece
of magical meanness." When the Kid speaks, he utters only
a magic code, "Coma ti yi youpy youpy yea." Coover sees
the idealized figure defined by a silence that adds to his
mystery and power. His potency resides as much in the others who fill the silence with a belief in his magical strength,
as in himself. Nobody else is allowed to speak his special
language. When the chorus tries to echo his doggerel, the
Kid's six-shooter riddles a poker game.

COWPOKE 44: Whew! I reckon he didn't like yuh shufflin them cards!

COWPOKE 45: Reckon he didn't like yuh breakin the silence!

COWPOKE 46: S-s-sorry, Kid!

COWPOKE 47: The Kid's big on silence!

COWPOKE 48: You said it, podnuh!

COWPOKE 49: *Very* big!

COWPOKE 50: The biggest.

The Kid contains a secret. He protects it by his impenetrable silence. The cowpokes are babblers who take their energy from the group. The Kid stands (and talks) alone. His mystery is translated into sexual fantasy. His prowess is extolled in magical terms. Belle Starr sings her story:

> They wasn't a cowboy in the whole blessed West
> That could stay in the saddle, I busted the best!
> But, boys lemme tell you, I got quite a surprise
> The day I got bestrid by the Kid with blue eyes. . . .

His penis, she discloses, is black and with a blue eye on the tip:

> Now, I've told yuh it's black with a little blue eye,
> But it's worse than that, boys, and I'll tell you why:
> It's also as cold as the stone of a tomb
> On a dead winter's night and it froze up muh womb!

In Coover's play, the Kid is gunned down by the Sheriff. The Sheriff becomes "the fastest gun in the West"; he's number one. After applauding his fast gun, the chorus of cowhands begin to refashion the Sheriff in the Kid's image —dressing him with the Kid's spurs and his "shootin' irons." The Sheriff is befuddled by this:

NO, DAMMIT, HOLD ON! . . . What I wanted tuh say was this. Somethin like this. Well, okay. It was me or the Kid. That's easy tuh folla. And the Kid got it. But . . . but it coulda jist as easy been me, see? No . . . no, that ain't it. That ain't exactly right. Whoo! Ifn I didn't know you boys better, I'd say yuh was tryin tuh get me drunk. See, what I'm tryin to tell yuh, boys, is they ain't no such thing as the fastest gun in the West. Yes! *That's* what I'm tryin tuh say! Me and the Kid there, see, it jist happened like. It don't mean a thing. . . .

The cowpokes want a transformation. They will a hero into being. The Deputy asks the Sheriff for the Kid's guns. As soon as he takes them out, they explode—as if by magic—and kill the Deputy. Violence becomes a self-fulfilling prophecy.

COWPOKE 212: Good gawdamighty! Did yuh see that!
COWPOKE 213: His own Deppity!
COWPOKE 214: Right between the fuckin eyes!
COWPOKE 215: Greased lightnin, man!
SHERIFF *(still in awe at his own hands)*: That . . . that's not what I—
COWPOKE 216 *(loud and commanding, as though suddenly taken aback)*: Whoa there! Hey! Stand back, you jaspers!
COWPOKE 217: Hunh?
COWPOKE 218: What the—!
COWPOKE 216 *(again)*: You see what I see?
COWPOKE 219 *(in overdrawn astonishment)*: Well, I'll be horn-swoggled! It ain't the Sheriff at all!
COWPOKE 220: The Kid!
COWPOKE 221: It's the Kid hisself!
COWPOKE 222: THE KID'S COME BACK!!

Despite the Sheriff's protests, the cowboys see what they

want to see. When the Sheriff throws down the silver pistols, they blast away as if they had a life of their own. The Sheriff throws off the Kid's garb and shouts his disclaimer, "You wouldn't lissen! Yuh wouldn't LISSEN tuh me!" The cowpokes need the myth more than the man. They kill the Sheriff to keep their notion of the Kid alive. The ambiguity Coover puts on stage is a modern spiritual predicament— man's need for mystery and also his fear of it. After lynching the Sheriff/Kid, the cowpokes return to their nostalgia for the magical experience he provided. The Kid's luminous aura is a fiction that evades their violence. Disliking paradoxes, the mind forges an impossible sense of coherence in the hero's destiny. The cowpoke chorus sings its final song about the Kid, triumphantly mixing fantasy and anticipation of impossible victory:

> He was mean, he was magic, he was real!
> Sweet Jesus, he was somethin tuh see!
> He was white as the lilies a the field
> And as pure and as wild and as free. . . .

Coover skewers the West that is preserved in its songs and extravagant figures. He also offers a theatrical event whose mystery lies in making concrete the vagaries of the imagination.

III

Mystery is obsessive; it haunts the imagination. Theater can be concocted with a phony elusiveness (Albee's *Tiny Alice*), where red herrings serve to jazz up humdrum plot lines. But when the mystery of language and the dynamics of the human mind are deeply felt by a playwright, his work exudes a resonance and truth. Too often, modern theater reflects the fear rather than the beauty of an obsession. For every Max and Lenny (in *The Homecoming*) who extend their mania to shattering, unpredictable gestures, there are hundreds of compromised Georges and Marthas (of *Who's Afraid of Virginia Woolf?*) who begin with the kernel of weirdness only to retreat from the dangerous consequences of unexpected actions.

John Ford Noonan's *The Year Boston Won the Pennant* deals with obsession—people locked into their private fantasies, with their own rules for survival. This is not a world of contrived riddles or arcane references. It is more real and harrowing. The tale centers around Marcus Sykowski, a once-famous pitching star on an odyssey in search of money for a new chrome arm with which to make a comeback. In his celebrity, Sykowski is the focus of many mysteries. Who is he? How did he lose his arm? As hero, people want him to explain the enigma of his personality. In a caddie pen where he earns money and builds up his remaining throwing arm, one of the regulars is infuriated by the simple seriousness of his determination. Marcus lifts a weighted bag. The other caddie, Jo Jo Delorenzo, circles around him, jabbing questions past the defense of silence.

> Jo Jo: Come on, how'd you ever blow the 75G's, what about what you made last year? And how come the management ain't supporting you, I mean, you're famous. Kid, come on. I gotta have something good to tell Momma, else— This is crazy! Didn't you even have insurance? . . .

Jo Jo receives no answers. He prods, insults, harangues—

but the mystery is not resolved. When Marcus leaves the caddie pen, pursued by a nameless man in a raincoat, Jo Jo lifts up Marcus's weighted bag. He, who scoffed at Marcus's comeback, feels the weight and suddenly, mysteriously believes. "He's gunna do it . . . gunna make it back with a metal arm. He told me so himself."

Noonan dramatizes uncertainty resolving itself in absolute faith. Marcus is a pitcher, aware only gradually of the importance people read into him. The world shapes men silently. Noonan understands the intangible pressures. The time of his play is just after a war has ended. People are frazzled, diminished by a violence which has never touched them. The essence of this modification is a mirror game where the discoveries of minor characters cast their reflections on the main character as well as on themselves. Marcus, for instance, is questioned by a soldier just back from the war. The dialogue is brittle and oblique, evoking in a few lines a world of cruelty and ignorance that haunts the play. The soldier, Miniver Peabody, says:

> I read in the paper some guy up in Maine, when he heard you got your arm chopped . . . went to bed and burned himself to death with gasoline . . . and with a monkey next to him no less. . . . Wow, were you well liked, huh?

Later in the same scene Miniver is suddenly gripped by despair. He questions Marcus about the Red Sox, whose destiny, without their ace pitcher, is in jeopardy. In his questions there is a hint of a larger void he can only vaguely articulate:

> All the time we were fighting the Kinks, all the way home on the ship, all we talked about was the Red Sox and how

they were a cinch for the pennant next year but now, now what's gunna happen to them, huh, now what's gunna happen?

He slams Marcus's stump and sends him to his knees in agony. The gesture and the need which brings it about are reminders of the ferocious and murky motivation behind every human action.

Noonan, like so many of the best contemporary dramatists, is not interested in the "becauses" of drama. He presents the audience with a series of events and a gallery of moral gargoyles. The future is conjecture, as is the past. Personality itself is paradox, a combination of the literal and the hidden, the surface and the submerged. Theatrical conventions of motivation, space, and time conjure the illusion of clarity. By disavowing them, Noonan emphasizes life's essential unpredictability, a mystery whose disturbing lapses of cohesion are filled by the mind and by myth.

Noonan's characters operate out of an unstated but carefully constructed emotional need. Their actions may be enough to take an audience by surprise; but, built on complex and deeply felt emotion, they cannot be dismissed as cerebral inventions. His people do not confront life as efficiently as they would in naturalistic theater. To be realistic about experience, the writer must take into account the silences, evasions, masks through which the human animal makes contact with the rest of his species. Noonan's dialogue exhibits an actor's understanding of human response: what people say is not necessarily what they mean. Mystery surrounds every process. Miniver shares an intimate dinner with his wife, Martha. This is his first night home. Soon Marcus will interrupt their ritual; but now

Martha is seized with obsessive laughter. "God bless these strange times when we can talk to what's going on inside of us," she then says to her husband with a confidence in rationality her dialogue (and the play) denies:

MARTHA: You're in a direct light. I can see the white of your scalp. . . .

MINIVER: It'll grow back. . . .

MARTHA *(pause, eating)* : It must have been the awful weather over there.

MINIVER: In the army you cut your hair short!

MARTHA *(pause, eating)* : There are globules of sweat running through your scalp. I can see them. *(Looking at each other, silence)* You're warm because your uniform's made of wool. *(Eating)* You look very handsome in it. *(Pause)* Do you ever think you'll take it off?

MINIVER: Soon. . . .

MARTHA: I was faithful while you were away.

MINIVER *(smiling)*: Yes. . . .

MARTHA *(eating)*: It confused me. . . . *(Suddenly another outburst of laughter)* Oh, why can't I control myself? Was it a regular thing thinking of me while you were away?

MINIVER *(long pause)*: Only when I was with a woman. . . .

MARTHA: Did it work?

MINIVER: Once. . . .

The submerged violence between Martha and Miniver springs out of madness masquerading as reason. The characters speak of moments of lost control as if their lives were totally ordered. The line between insanity and intelligence is shortened. Noonan's tactic refuses an audience its passive role as a witness to packaged formulas. Through mystery, the stage aspires not to a slice of life but to the elusive clarity of dream. The audiences must concentrate on each individual moment. They do not judge; they experience.

In *The Year Boston Won the Pennant,* Marcus is pursued by
the Man in the Raincoat, a henchman connected to the
forces who have maimed him, and a theatrical descendant
of Rosencrantz and Guildenstern via Goldberg and
McCann. In his play people watch people, just as in life the
CIA and FBI keep files. This pursuit is also symbolic, dramatizing the national obsession for public as well as private
verification. As a national hero Marcus is constantly being
asked to explain himself. Omnipresent in Noonan's play are
references to newspapers and television, social forces incul-
cating a false sense of "objectivity" and the right of the public to know all. Speaking at the graveside of Gyles Lurt-
sema, the boy who has immolated himself after learning of
Marcus's injury, Marcus can only explain his pitching as
magic ("When you're pouring rhythm sweet, when you got
it, really got it . . . they can't see it, they can't smell it,
can't touch it, can't even believe it . . . cause it's yours . . .
it's magic!"). He cannot understand why people are so passionate about his life and why they press him for explanations:

> MARCUS: I read the Boston papers all the way up here. . . .
> They want to know what's going to happen to me, Gyles,
> what's to happen to my wind-up, my kick, my great bal-
> ance. They say "Why doesn't he take help from the Red
> Sox . . . for what reason did he refuse the insurance aid,
> what about the wife and child? They say, the papers, they
> think I should say to the police how my arm was
> chopped, that as a great and known figure of America I
> owe it . . .

Mystery allows fluidity on stage. Nothing is certain, and
this underscores the insanity behind the other characters'

furious sense of rational purpose. If Marcus is a real hero and almost a center of worship, Noonan shows technology at work creating synthetic idols. Candy Cane, Marcus's wife, is pushed into revealing a fake kidnaping over national television, using her husband's name and the national exposure to launch her movie career. Leroy Star, who has conceived the plot, understands the purpose and power of the medium. It offers a new mythology, instant belief which emasculates the figures it raises up for "worship." The media give a sense of purpose and an illusion of logic to the world. As Star explains:

> Our America's upside down, Honey, people tromp around in tears, their heads jangling with fire. Our wondrous citizens are lost and I tell you why. All the big names dead, gone, they got nothing to look up to, no new personalities, no celebrated stars. I'm using you to save our America, to raise its hope and head. . . .

The irony is that often it is the cynosural figures of our society who hide the truth from it. They deny mystery, an experience which negates the sense of direction their images imply. At the end Marcus is shot on the pitching mound at Fenway Park. He has always believed in the system which promoted him but which must also destroy him. Noonan's play, like Coover's, dramatizes the paradox of the public imagination: the public annihilates what it cannot absorb or explain.

The Year Boston Won the Pennant gives us a world which has completely forgotten the vagaries of creation, which has been brainwashed by an efficient capitalism and become numb to its own logical violence. The play dramatizes the destiny of insanity R. D. Laing has prophesied for modern man:

In order to rationalize our industrial-military complex, we have to destroy our capacity to see clearly any more what is in front of, and to imagine what is beyond, our noses. Long before a thermonuclear war can come about, we have had to lay waste our sanity.[11]

The stage event is public dream, but the American theater has forgotten the importance of what Jung called "fantastic thinking." [12] Mystery frees the theater from the shackles of literalism. It gives modern theater a flexibility and a way of dealing with an artistic problem that Artaud defined:

> The question, then, for the theater, is to create a metaphysics of speech, gesture, and expression, in order to rescue it from its servitude to psychology and "human interest." But all this can be of no use unless behind such an effort there is some kind of real metaphysical inclination, an appeal to certain unhabitual ideas, which by their very nature cannot be limited or even formally depicted.[13]

Theater loses its energy when it caters to bourgeois intentions. Stability, comfort, safety are middle-class maxims that deny the life of the stage as well as the soul. Audiences are "uncomfortable" around complexity, but it is when the theater zeros in on life that the experience becomes painful and important. On stage, mystery is both dangerous and thrilling. Existing between the extremes of outrage and silence, mystery affirms the coexistence of the external world with an inner one, the material with the spiritual. Mystery forces modern theater back to a humanity it has almost forgotten and an integrity of inquiry whose resources it is just learning to tap.

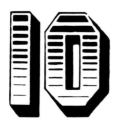

Heathcote Williams' *AC/DC*:
Flushing the Toilet
in the Brain

The images the mass media convey cross all
boundaries, local and national, permit each
individual everywhere to be overwhelmed by
superficial messages and undigested cultural
elements, but at the same time often cause
him to be overwhelmed by superficial
messages and undigested cultural elements,
by headlines and by endless partial
alternatives.
  —Robert J. Lifton, *Boundaries*

AC/DC is about the victims of historical velocity. Heathcote Williams' phenomenal play takes the television set as
the central symbol of our technological age—an object in
which our passion for speed and obsession with energy coalesce. Ours is the moment, as radio stations brag, of "all-in-

formation-all-the-time," and the medium of television feeds our craving the way Dr. Faustus's magic carpet served his insatiable appetite for knowledge and power. Flooded with imagery, modern man is isolated from events yet always conscious of them. He feels powerless in a universe that seems at his fingertips.

The new generation's desire to change shape is a survival tactic. No writer epitomizes and re-creates the anguish and visionary longing of this protean generation better than Williams, who admits to "feelings of extreme impotence and extreme inability to control one's environment." [1] Although Williams is British, his play speaks more accurately to the exaggerations of the American media. *AC/DC*—a title incorporating transformation and energy sources—synthesizes and clarifies deep areas of psychic dislocation in the culture. The play depicts the sensory overload. Its style is the same bombardment of information and ideas that makes Williams' claim that "the human animal is totally convertible" [2] not only logical but necessary. *AC/DC* is a "brain-buzz," a bypass circuit for "media rash" which gives shape and definition to the behavioral effects of media static. Williams explains:

> Electro-magnetic pollution is not just an allegory for psychic manipulation: it's physical. In *Time* magazine, October 26, 1970, I read an extraordinary article in which mischief-making radio waves had been held responsible for opening electrically operated garage doors, and where stray waves from micro-wave ovens had stopped pacemakers designed to steady the beat of a faltering heart. Perhaps Maurice is a schizophrenic character. But whereas a few years ago in order to pick up electric signals in the brain it was necessary to drill a tiny hole in the skull and insert a platinum needle; now signals can be picked up simply by putting on a sort of

hair-dryer stashed with electrodes over one's head. If signals can be picked up outside the brain, it's not too far-fetched a contention to suggest that all this electronic smog is penetrating the brain as well. *All the characters are trying to do some housework: they're trying to clean up their brains. They've all been plunged into a giant electronic whispering gallery. They're trying to regulate their infective thresholds; and if they can't do it, they'll seal them off.*[3] (my italics)

Williams is defining man's spiritual odyssey as he adapts to a technological society. But the call for a new man to cope with new energy goes back much further. In 1905, the historian Henry Adams found the symbol of the new industrial age in the Dynamo. In one chapter of his *Autobiography*, "The Dynamo and the Virgin," Adams prophesies the psychic shift of the culture from the regenerative spiritual force (the Virgin) to physical force (the Dynamo). Looking out at the sky line of New York, Adams felt "an absolute fiat in electricity as in faith."[4] In the high combustion of twentieth-century America, life would never be the same:

Power seemed to have outgrown its servitude and to have asserted its freedom. The cylinder had exploded and thrown great masses of stone and steam against the sky. . . . Prosperity never before imagined, power never reached by anything but a meteor, had made the world irritable, nervous, querulous, unreasonable and afraid. All New York was demanding new men, and all the new forces, condensed into corporations, were demanding a new type of man—a man with ten times the endurance, energy, will and mind of the old type—for whom they were willing to pay millions at first sight. . . .[5]

In its energy and promise of progress, the Dynamo was the highest mechanical embodiment of pioneer will power. The Dynamo focused not on deepening the inner landscape

but on transforming the external one. This created a spiritual vacuum. Television attempts to fill this vacuum and
symbolizes the exhaustion and superficiality of man's impetus in the world. Confronted by the failure of his will, man
seeks escape in fantasy. Ninety-five per cent of American
homes have television sets, twenty-five per cent of these
homes have two or more. Between the ages of two and sixty-
five, the average male viewer will spend 3000 days—nine
full years of life—gazing at the phosphorescent images.[6]

At a certain momentum, matter disintegrates. Technology has pushed the society to a relentless velocity where,
without any redemptive ideal, it seeks the balm of total release in the fantasy of television. A nation which once
dreamed of itself as dynamic has turned into a nation of
amnesiacs.

In Adams' description of the New Man, the individual
subordinated his will to the machine. Williams' polymor-
phic man must change his terms of reference to protect
himself from a domineering technology. Transformation is
his rallying cry. His search is for new imagery and new energy on the path toward symbolic immortality. Frantic and
schizoid from the collision of his potential self with the one
conditioned by society, his fight is a life-and-death struggle.
Protean man wants a resurrection, but not at the mercy of
the machine. He wants to tap his own inner resources. Hal-
lucinogens provide an inner imagery intended to be a transcendence. He "blows his mind," gets "wasted," or "freaks
out." The terms for his "changes" are not only those of destruction, but of a conscious mutation. Taking a trip is a
schizoid tactic to straight-arm the sense of suffocation which
television compounds in the culture. Perowne, a terminal
schizophrenic in *AC/DC* whose immense potential is para-

lyzed by the media overload, stares at the television and announces his revenge:

America should be put to sleep for a hundred years. America's a psychopath. But psychopaths can still deploy themselves. They can still make strategies, they can still make very careful plots. The thing to do is not to try and check it, but to Continue the parameter. To combat irrationality with irrationality. To make it entirely schizophrenic. Properly schizophrenic. *(Holding out his hand as if holding a gun. An American accent)* How am I expected to fire this gun, when it looks like a cabbage? HEY MACK, I CAN'T FIRE THIS GUN, THE TRIGGER'S STARTED MENSTRUATING.

Perowne advocates madness as a strategy for survival, a tactic which Americans have witnessed in a more decorative way with the Beats, the Hippies, the Yippies *et al.* Williams explores madness as energy on stage as a possible means of approaching the divine.

"In reading case histories of schizophrenia," says Williams, "I've come across many references by patients to electrical interference to their peace of mind, and the feeling that electricity was somehow responsible for their movements and attitudes." [7] Now, with television, the schizophrenic's complaint of "wires in the head" is metaphorically, if not literally, true. Every $\frac{1}{30}$th of a second a new electron image is produced on the screen. Television creates a "global village" where the viewer is forever on the outskirts. Dr. Eugene D. Glynn has claimed that television is "schizoid fostering" and "smothers contact, really inhibiting personal exchange." [8] The viewer knows what's happening and yet nothing confronts him. Television traps the viewer in someone else's dream—either the government's or the advertiser's or the star's. Hungry for distraction and too resourceless to fight back, the average viewer passively consents to this suffocation. But in *AC/DC* the problem is dramatized by people striking back:

> If you detect a flavor of the black arts in the play, this is again one of their solutions: Sadie's at any rate. It comes from feelings of isolation, as witches always existed in isolated communities. . . . There is no transistor in the circuit with her name on it. She has no access to decision-making machinery, so she switches the terms of reference entirely to escape the machine, to prevent it from recognizing her.[9]

The Dynamo represented the anticipation of abundance. Television is a means of coping with the betrayal of that dream of benevolence. People turn to television as if to sympathetic magic, but television compromises the play instinct. In front of the tube, the self is comatose. Doctors are now encountering what they call "T.V. spine" and "T.V. eyes." [10] Filtering other people's fantasies, the mind has neither the time nor silence to probe. The self becomes a shut-in. Television offers the false omnipotence of fantasy in a society where so much is promised and so little delivered. The video cassette will aggravate this by allowing the viewer to pre-empt the already managed news by his special taste for escape.

Television coaxes the viewer into expectations of psychic wholeness.[11] We know more, therefore we should be more. But, through television, the split between mind and body is widened. The speed and multiplicity of images eliminates the spectator's imaginative work and also blurs his spiritual /historical memory. With television our memory is debilitated because we do not discover, but are shown.

We recall the past not only by recording it but by reliving it, by making present again its fears and delectations. We anticipate the future not only by preparing for it but by conjuring up and creating it. Our links to yesterday and tomorrow depend also on the aesthetic, emotional, and symbolic aspects of human life—on saga, play, and celebration.[12]

AC/DC touches our past and shows us a future. As Sadie observes of Maurice, the play "is satirizing ideas that haven't yet arisen."

I

SADIE: . . . I don't mind having a few psychic capitalists inside my head when I'm eating, if that's where they want to be, or even when I'm fucking, but to have that Grade-B tinsel-town shit batting round in my head when I'm fixin' to DIE . . . No man, no, no, no. . . .

    —*AC/DC* (II)

The "tinsel-town shit" is the psychic clutter served up by our junk culture. The imagery of stars, films, incidental data plays back through the brain and creates a mosaic which constitutes our "inner life." This imagery is the residue of our passion for distraction. It represents a means by which we evade our suffering and any profound understanding of ourselves. In this condition, the self is imprisoned. The human will is stymied by a festering, general malaise. Unless suffering can be faced and worked through, the spirit is strangled and mauled by a despair which, because it is unexamined, cannot be turned to life-giving enlightenment. Like the characters in *AC/DC*, Williams is trying "to fight [his] way out of a clogged psychic environment: where's the toilet in my brain, how do I flush it?" [13]

AC/DC dramatizes an act of renewal in which the self absorbs suffering and is led to a deeper understanding of human experience. Williams' evocation of the struggle for transcendence in *AC/DC* is an answer to the malevolent, uncreative suffering he depicted in his first one-act play, *The Local Stigmatic*. There, the will is frustrated and destructive. Suffering finds its expression in revenge. Adrift in the world, starved of relationships, trusting anybody who speaks with authority, Williams' two central characters—Graham and Ray—are from a culture of spectators. They read the papers and the fan magazines; they talk about the winners in the world as well as at the dog track. They are psychopaths—without historical memory and without guilt. Strangers to themselves, their sense of loss finds its expression in mockery. Graham and Ray can't protect themselves from the allure of the "psychic capitalists" of *AC/DC*. Graham and Ray are invisible figures in a technological society that puts a premium on visibility. They are enchanted by the famous, and also destroyed by them. At the pub, they meet a star and chat him up. Their object of reverence—David—is shown to be hollow and vain. David's will is foisted upon them through publicity. Their anger at this bondage takes the form of annihilation. Graham and Ray ask David for his autograph. They walk him home. They set him up, and then maim him. Graham talks while Ray, having thrown a coat over David's head, works what he calls "the old black magic." Violence gives them a sense of power; it lets them feel real emotion.

> GRAHAM: . . . No, David, let's put it another way for you. It's the simplest thing in the world when you grasp it. You

see, take Ray for example . . . this girl Sharon that he's shacked up with: *she* thinks he's *you* and when they're in bed, David, *he* thinks he's you, and she thinks she's been done by you, you see. Now, it's not quite as simple as you think. . . . Kick him again Ray, keep at it. . . . You see, David, it's got nothing to do with RESENTING you, nothing at all . . . it's just that it seems stupid that you're not THERE to defend yourself, you see . . .

David, like all Sadie's psychic capitalists in *AC/DC*, has sold himself into the minds of millions. Graham and Ray live with him on their brains, and now he will live with the memory of them. But, even in this violent bludgeoning, they continue to live in other people's rhythms, finding energy not in themselves but in others. They decide to call David on the phone six months after the punch-up:

GRAHAM: Give him a ring.
RAY: It's ex-directory.
GRAHAM: Belgravia two one five six. Use your Douglas Fairbanks voice, Ray.

Graham and Ray are shadows: imitation is their only possible act. They mime the world that destroys them. Who's winning? What's happening? They are riveted to the surface of events. They observe the world with an insatiable curiosity and fear; but without the resources to go inside themselves.

AC/DC answers the perversity of this psychic state. Here, the characters are clearly focused on interior experience. Williams presents five people on different spiritual rungs on the ladder to self-awareness. Itinerants of the Hip world, Gary and Melody use the recipes of drugs, sex, mysticism for diversion, not discovery. Sadie, their friend, is looking for a more serious breakthrough. She wants a more profound reality and knows that "reality at white heat is holiness." Maurice contains the energy to push himself into new shapes and approach the divine. He turns his schizophrenic suffering to creative use, absorbing the static in Perowne's head and reaching new spheres of understanding. At the beginning, Maurice exists on a higher wave length than the rest; but eventually, Perowne, with Sadie's help, surpasses him. Perowne, a man capable of breaking psychic boundaries, is paralyzed by sensory overload: "I don't know. I don't know if it's too late. The sensory assault is too great. It's really a stress situation." Williams' characters all share the same problem: how to clear the mind's congestion and renew authentic energy by deepening a sense of self. *AC/DC* astonishes with its gift of prophecy and the intellectual conviction with which Williams dramatizes the metaphysical struggle to attain a higher semantic-emotional-cognitive stratum.

II

In truth, man is a polluted river. One must be
a sea to receive a polluted river and not be
defiled.

 —NIETZSCHE, *Thus Spake Zarathustra*

AC/DC's first act—Alternating Current—is set against the frenetic, abrasive energy field of a penny arcade. At Playland, electronic energy is running riot. "Ball bearings churn and wheep through the bumpers" of pinball machines. The circuitry is a symbolic extension of our nervous system, and Maurice, the repairman, also knows how to put things right in the mind. The wild, frantic discharges of the arcade—its flashing neon, its banked television sets blinking multiangled pictures of the audience back at it—epitomizes the electronic mayhem and disorientation of the minds congregated at Playland. The characters, like the current, make occasional contact, while yearning for some fluid connection, a transcendent consciousness to fend off the intensity of the media mosaic and bring peace. The adventurous quality of all these technological mutants is apparent from their first "spaced" dialogue as flashbulbs from the Photomaton pop to record their latest odyssey.

> GARY: MONGOLIAN CLUSTER FUCK!
> MELODY: YEAAAAH! KICKED OUT ALL THE PHYSICAL JAMS!
> GARY: GLUED US ALL TOGETHER!
> SADIE: THREE IN ONE AND ONE IN THREE!

They talk of "mind-swaps" and "changes," they long to be transformed and reborn. "Healed all the crimps," says Melody. "Hey, we really laid some changes on each other, no? I feel completely Burst, completely Deconditioned. Just like I been doing some astral projections and I just slipped back into my body this second and it's a perfect fit." The static in this environment is not merely electric, but psychic. People are trying to cross-circuit each other, to get into each other's trips. From the beginning, language itself becomes a means of reviving the mind to make spiritual leaps. Maurice is the focus of energy in this environment. He is the schizophrenic as hero, a psychic superman, whose verbal and spiritual aura can turn minds upside down. He protects his lover, Perowne, from electronic radiation and media fallout. Pulling at his scalp, Maurice boasts:

> . . . And this is where three phrenologists lost their fingernails. In me riah. In me fuckin barnet. And five years ago, they shaved it all off, pasted wires on, and plugged me into their so-called amnesiac shockers. But I broke the box, and fused every light in the area for thirty miles.

In the first act, Gary and Melody are using Sadie as their energy source. This is how they are grouped on stage; and how, in acting terms, their need is expressed. Maurice and Perowne are on another circuit, a direct current. As Maurice explains, "What's going on between Perowne and me is peak to peak amplitude." Nobody can break into Maurice's high frequency. Perowne explains Maurice's linguistic strategy:

> Maurice does it. He does it in the way he talks. Cholinergic. Adrenergic. Shamanistic. He closes down their transmissions. He generates such an amount of psychic static that they can't get through.

Sadie is attracted to Maurice's high energy. She understands what he's doing. She is hungry for a fuller identity, and there is a voraciousness in her playful wrestling with Maurice. *"They growl at each other, and then roll over each other on the floor grappling and laughing."* The stage directions indicate a new emotional alignment. "MAURICE *and* SADIE *collapse breathless under the Photomaton.* GARY *and* MELODY *move across to one of the pinmachines. Beat Time."* Watching Maurice perform with Perowne convinces Sadie how shallow and tame her explorations have been with Melody and Gary. The physical separation of the characters on stage underscores their mental breach. Melody and Gary try to discredit Maurice, but they cannot follow where he leads. Sadie denounces them. Melody and Gary steal the jargon of a Hip world, but lack the courage to battle the culture. Theirs is a revolt of style, not mind. By avoiding suffering, they evade themselves.

Sadie, like Maurice, begins to use language as an energy vector, a sexual act of penetration. Maurice, who is touched by every electronic vibration, uses language as the outlet for this absorption of energy.

> MAURICE: Perowne filled my teeth in a certain way, you see, certain alloys in certain combinations, so that I was picking up tv programmes in my head like a Jew's Harp, and he shoved David Niven-Richard-Harris-Hemmings-Photo-down my head very hard and, switching my body clock on, off, on, off, and every time I kissed Perowne I was forced to desalivate because of course Perowne didn't want David Niven's style of kissing. . . .

Maurice feels and conquers the energy. He finds great sources of power in himself. Perowne does not. He's stymied and tortured by the intake. The imagery does visceral damage to him. He has not found a way, like Maurice, of focusing the energy. He does not, like Maurice, feel his mind and body working as a unified force. He is petrified and confounded. He over-amps.

> PEROWNE: . . . I've been watching a lot of television.
> MAURICE: You've got fuckin radiated, haven't you? You've got fuckin media rash, haven't you?

PEROWNE: Well, I watched the news. The television. You
see. I watched the news *(twitching)*. Then I went into the
street. Whole place is a noisy ashtray. . . .

The audience, like the characters, absorbs a new and totally sustained verbal onslaught. The language of technology and force, which dominates the external world, is the
most accurate expression of spiritual suffering.

MAURICE: . . . Every word I utter is the radioactive waste of
eighteen million telepathons. Every word that's pumped
through me is eighteen million telepathons down the
drain. I don't want to use words.

Words stream out of each character's mouth. Affected by
so much in the world, these protean people speak a language which registers the multiplicity of impulses. Speech
acts like a magnetic field, attracting ideas, motives, trivia,
resonances. The density of the dialogue gives Williams'
characters an unusual theatrical complexity. Williams says:

Character as usually portrayed on stage is hopelessly stratified. There are millions of things batting around inside
your head that will remain undisclosed until there is direct
brain to brain contact. You tell me a story now and tomorrow I tell the story to somebody else. Who's this somebody
else listening to, you or me? He's actually listening to a
group mind. I would like to be able to convey the nature of
this psychic static: the unnamed and unarticulated con-
tracts that exist between two human beings in dialogue: this
background noise like the drone of a universal bagpipe.[14]

III

Man is something that should be overcome.
What have you done to overcome him?

—NIETZSCHE, *Thus Spake Zarathustra*

The second act—Direct Current—takes place in Perowne's room. The space is as cluttered as his cranium. Red and yellow wires climb around the walls like ganglia; television sets are banked around the room flashing new imagery every second to compete with over 2000 glossy photographs of the Famous which paper the walls. Williams' second environment is as overwhelming and brilliant as the first. In this hypnotic space, there is no possibility of living firsthand. Discovery, and, therefore, growth, become impossible because the viewer must be passive to receive the stimulation. Images of good and evil, purity and debasement have the same visual weight and impact. Perowne dreams of revenge on a television newsman. His fantasy comes to him over the video screens. The television is his mind; his mind is the television. He confronts the newsreader's wife at her home and protests about her husband's performance.

> . . . You see your husband's technique involves the theft of a facial expression that he used on the Middle East crisis, for announcing the cricket scores. And the Middle East gets this facial expression back, because your husband is ashamed of being found out. So the cricket scores are then of exactly the same weight to the Middle East crisis.

In Perowne's exaggerations, Williams makes important criticism of the effects of the media on the mind. Events blur in their speed; battles and ball games, moonshots and market reports come to us with the same audiovisual impact. A nation's behavioral patterns—its violence, its consumer needs, its language—are silently transformed by the routine of television. Perowne wants to get beyond the borrowed energy of his room. The Famous are beamed in front of him every second. They constitute a pseudohistory, and television fosters a bogus intimacy between the viewer and the viewed. Perowne needs them and hates himself for this impossible love in which his care is wasted.

> PEROWNE: . . . They're stealing one's instinctual patterns. THEY'RE STEALING THEM. THEY'RE FORGING THEM. THEY'RE SLOWING THEM UP. THEY'RE SPEEDING THEM UP. THEY'RE REPRODUCING THEM TWENTY TIMES A DAY. THEY'RE UN-LOADING YOU. THEY'RE OVERLOADING YOU. . . .

"Fame," Williams says, "is the perversion of the natural instinct for validation and attention." [15] Television provides a means for instant celebrity; and, as every mother knows, a surrogate for personal contact. This fosters a devastating sense of impotence. The invisible public lives through the synthetic energy of their visible stars. Perowne, as he moves further into himself and away from the world, is a victim of this death-dealing media dependence. Celebrity replaces history. Williams has said:

> As the media stand now .0001 per cent of the population is getting *crème brûlée* every day, and the rest are being ignored. Without attention our feedback system breaks down because we don't know who we are. With too much of it you turn into a completely different being—what is called in the play a psychic capitalist. And it's dangerous that the landscape is arranged by a minority. I was in favor of the Yippies breaking up David Frost's programme, because Frost is like a ruthless bank manager saying, "This is my event; all the vibrations in this room belong to me." [16]

Perowne's media affliction reduces him to infantile postures. He crawls, stands on his chair, sits in catatonic silence. His actions symbolize the emotional condition to which the viewer is reduced. Television's nickname, "the glass tit," is apt. Speaking of the social effects of broadcasting, Gerhart Wiebe has pointed out the parallel between viewing and child behavior. "The media" offer immediate need gratification without "paying the piper. . . ." The media allow the audience to resume the infantile posture observed by Piaget in which, when stimulus is removed, it ceases to exist. . . ." [17]

When Sadie enters Perowne's room, she has come to test the transcendental superiority of her energy. Perowne is the litmus paper of her experiment. Sadie is forced to compete with Maurice for Perowne. Williams sets up the moment cunningly. Maurice has been flexing his psychic muscle for Perowne, recounting with hilarious gusto his run-in with and victory over R. D. Laing.

> MAURICE: I DID MORE THAN THAT! PSYCHIATRY PSYCHOLOGY of any Good is about LOVE. Getting Close to People through LOVE, and anything that falls short of that is no Good. And he was 17,000 protein holograms short of LOVE. Fancy starting a love affair with "Totalisations of your cathectic meta-selves. . . ."

Perowne is begging for Maurice's energy to neutralize the television imagery: "THEY'RE ALTERING MY NEURAL RHYTHMS. THEY'RE PULLING THEM INTO SYNCH WITH THEIR NEURAL RHYTHMS. THEY'RE CODING ALL MY CELLS. WHAT ARE YOU GOING TO DO ABOUT IT? . . ." Perowne taunts Sadie to "prove her vibrations." The moment is right for a contest. Sadie must prove herself to Perowne; and, to sustain the audience's credibility in his gift of prophecy, Williams must produce an act of stage magic powerful enough to match the high-amperage energy of her claim. He succeeds in one of the most brilliant scenes in modern English drama.

Sadie sizes up Perowne's room and realizes that the images must be stripped away. She knows that Perowne was formerly an IBM researcher and so she puts her diagnosis into cybernetic terms. The room is a flow chart: "Input, see, autocorrelation, anticipatory feedback. . . . A Cybernetic Time Series of Sign Stimuli releasing adaptive patterns of behavior *(pointing to the wall)* then . . . OUTPUT! *(Pointing to* PEROWNE*)* and AFFECT!"

Sadie gets into Perowne's head. The idea of a cybernetic model captures Perowne's imagination. Sadie leads him to a deeper understanding about the dilution of energy, the "scatter" of ideas and images which create psychic confusion. This spiritual quest unfolds with a gorgeous, riveting clarity.

PEROWNE: I did . . . I did half think of it as a cybernetic model. Let's see who you've . . . let's see who you've got in Input Section. Marilyn Monroe.

SADIE: Yeah, she's Input. She's Basic Basic.

PEROWNE *(pointing to the right, tracing a line)*: But then the Rot sets in. A kind of inverse Doppler effect. The original imprint is defaced, and you get Forty randomised functions trying to restimulate a need that's already been exhausted by Marilyn Monroe . . .

SADIE: THAT'S RIGHT! *(Pointing to the wall)* Carroll Baker, Sandra Milo, Anita Ekberg, Virna Lisi, Sharon Tate, Edie Adams, Barbara Loden, Kathy Kirby, Diana Dors, Jayne Mansfield . . .

PEROWNE: Servo-mechanisms which tend to over-correct the whole mechanism (to conceal their origins) so that the Whole Mechanism no longer proceeds towards the target area, but performs a series of lateral zig zags and eventually stops all forward progress all together . . . You get the . . . same thing here, I suppose—Input section, you get . . . *(pointing at a photo)* Wittgenstein. . . . Pure . . . then *(tracing a line with his finger through the photos)* then the breakdown of the original imprint into random functions . . . Random noise.

SADIE: . . . Look at it. Ha. *(She sways in front of the wall)* Ha. ALL THE PSYCHIC CAPITALISTS IN ONE GHETTO! *(Turning round to PEROWNE)* There's gotta be economy, no? Who's running the economy?

PEROWNE: YES. A lot of the circuitry's overloaded, and I find it . . . *(twisting)* I find it . . .

SADIE: Solid! There's gotta be some economy. Look at it *(closer to the wall)* Tom Jones . . . see? Cooked-down version of Sam Cook and Otis Redding. *(Tears down the photo of Tom Jones)* Bye bye Thomas. *(Studying the wall)* How many times does Donovan go into Bob Dylan? Bye bye Donovan. *(Tears down photo)* How many times does Dylan go into Woody Guthrie? *(Tears down photo)* Bye Bye Dylan . . . Elvis Presley, sanforised version of Arthur "Big Boy" Crudup. *(Tears down photo)* Marshall McLuhan, Readers Digest version of William Burroughs. Bye bye Marshall. *(Tears down photo. Moves along the wall)* Here's Fletcher Henderson, still being fraudulently restimulated by Benny Goodman. So long Bennie. . . .

Most of the pictures are stripped off the wall. The imagery is decontaminated and the energy they absorbed from Perowne gradually restored in him. The television is pissed on and massaged with a magnet to distort the electronic waves. Sadie is steering Perowne into deeper spiritual waters. To find images which are Basic Basic is one of the clues to spiritual liberation. Sadie shows Perowne that he must focus energy on resonant symbols, not squander it on false ones:

> THINK Perowne, what fuckin circuits would have come up if you could have stolen the Beatlemachine's energy. I mean: REAL BRAIN TO BRAIN CONTACT, instead of exhausting the energy need for that by selling the same Fake Chauvinistic Sex Bonds *(chanting)* Ooo-ooO OOH Love Me Do I Love You . . . Love ME do? . . .

Perowne's self is not something he has to guard like property from the omnivorous forces around him. By helping him block the imagery, Sadie guides Perowne to a sense of spiritual freedom. As theologian H. A. Williams writes:

> When we regard self as some limited entity which we possess and must guard, then what we possess in fact possesses us. We are not free to do what we like, for we must for ever be concerned with protecting our property. . . . So are we possessed by the self we consider ourselves to possess. It hinders us from being what we are and so from giving ourselves. We are its prisoners. . . . In these circumstances what suffering does is to destroy the house so that we have to find our home in the limitless spaces of the world. . . .[18]

With Sadie as a more creative catalyst, Perowne abandons Maurice as his psychic guardian. Maurice can clear the sensory overload, but he cannot channel Perowne's positive energy. Up to Perowne's break with Maurice, Perowne has used his friend as an evasion of suffering. With Sadie, he accepts suffering and goes beyond it. This is dramatized when Perowne goes into a planned epileptic spasm in front of the television, a maneuver which shows Sadie how much energy Perowne can marshal.

PEROWNE: . . . I can float anything I want into it and burn them into cancerous dust.

SADIE: Sheeeeit! That's the Heat Death of the Universe. You didn't tell me about that. . . . That's your Private By-Pass Circuit . . . you could wipe anything off the slate with that, no?

Maurice tries to elbow Sadie off the scene: "I was told the only cure for schizophrenia was to make at least two other people schizophrenic. I've sent Tuffnell up the pictures, so that only leaves one to go. What's your feeling about that?" But Sadie won't be bluffed. She is already beyond Maurice's spiritual wave length. Perowne's strategy is to exact punishment from the television. Sadie shows Perowne that he must turn the destructive will to a creative one; moving away from objects in the world toward some higher spiritual connection. She leads Perowne into a new emotional orbit where he is prepared to take the most radical action: to change himself, not society.

IV

. . . ready for lightning in its dark bosom
and for redeeming beams of life, pregnant
with lightnings which affirm Yes! laugh Yes!
ready for prophetic lightning flashes. . . .

—NIETZSCHE, *Thus Spake Zarathustra*

Schizoid energy is the consummate anarchist ideal. "If I could turn you on, if I could drive you out of your wretched mind. If I could tell you I would let you know." R. D. Laing's famous incantation in *The Politics of Experience* is echoed by Nietzsche's Superman, by Artaud's manifestos for a Theater of Cruelty. Madness is suggested as a path to wisdom. To break all boundaries, to refuse to communicate with an untenable world and move inward to deeper mythic sources, to mutate oneself and the universe, to drop out of historical time, and, denying gravity, to aspire to some visionary light, has become a cultural longing which *AC/DC* defines more profoundly than any theater piece of the generation. Artaud's schizoid fantasy of a Theater of Cruelty never created a stage work equal to his dream of transcendent energy which he likened to the plague and which:

> causes the masks to fall, reveals the lie, the slackness, the baseness and hypocrisy of the world; it shakes off the asphyxiating inertia of matter which invades even the clearest testimony of the senses; and in revealing to collectivities of men their dark power, *their hidden force*, it invites them to take, in face of destiny, a superior and heroic attitude they would never have assumed without it.[19] (my italics)

In the intensity and proportion of the psychic struggle, *AC/DC* assumes the heroic dimensions Artaud wrote about but never achieved.

LSD, Yoga, mystic spells are all evoked (and abandoned) by Maurice, Sadie, and Perowne as formulas for plunging inward. Joseph Campbell wrote in his essay "Schizophrenia—the Inward Journey" that with all these methods, "the range of visions experienced are, in fact, the same as those of psychosis." [20] Williams' stage schizophrenics exist in contrast to the schizoid suffocation of the media. They are grounded, like Williams himself, by extraordinary intellects which keep their transformations from becoming plastic adaptations.

AC/DC puts the real schizophrenic juice on stage. When Maurice discusses R. D. Laing, Williams is able to criticize the conventional "popularized" conception of the schizophrenic as hero. Williams' criticism of Laing is not that he is extreme but that he does not go far enough. Maurice wants the energy, the "juice" as he calls it. His imaginary hectoring of Laing is side-splitting: "You've got nothing. All you've got is a bit of polari picked up from a couple of half-chat existentialists and ex-wobblies." Besides the satire, Williams' criticism of Laing broadens the notion of the authentic schizophrenic experience.

> MAURICE *(nods)*: "Well, what started it off," he said. Well doctor I said. It doesn't feel like me talking. It's not me talking. And I've got to get rid of it, haven't I? *(Winking at* PEROWNE*)* It's a pony-tail haircut inside me talking.
> PEROWNE: That must have touched him where he liked it.
> MAURICE: . . . Stop trying to verb me up, because what you say doesn't last any longer than the length which you take to say it. Whereas, what I say, I'm converting into protein molecules, tied to the backs of neutrinos, going Straight through you and coming out the other side. I had your mind in 1935, and it was a messy little fuck then. . . . "The concept of cure," he said. "Is very outmoded." CURE? I want the juice. . . .
> . . . And all the time Perowne, he's marching round the inside of my head, grabbing every bit of electricity he can lay his hands on.
> PEROWNE: Stealing his patients' best ideas to give his trips a little local colour.
> MAURICE: THAT'S YOUR MAN! He's the root virus. He's the terminal Adjustive psychologist. But he still doesn't acknowledge them . . . his bastard patients are put down as "D" or "F.M." Or Occasionally "Arthur," whereas his own name comes up fifteen times in the credits.

> "Oh, so you've read my books?" he said.
> "I read your books at source . . ."

In some primitive cultures, schizophrenic terror is considered beneficial, and the "victim" becomes the shaman, the
high priest, who through his suffering has returned with
greater wisdom. In more rationally ordered cultures, the
emotional support is absent and the schizophrenic typically
undergoes an intensification of suffering over and above his
original anxieties.[21] But the shaman, the mystic, and the
schizophrenic share a crucial pattern; at their most profound, they die into life. Joseph Campbell writes:

> When the return or remission occurs, it is experienced as a
> rebirth: the birth, that is to say, of a "twice-born" ego, no
> longer bound in by its daylight-world horizon. It is now
> known to be but the reflex of a larger self, its proper func-
> tion being to carry the energies of an archetypal instinct sys-
> tem in fruitful play in a contemporary space-time daylight
> situation.[22]

Williams' final image in *AC/DC* evokes this yearning for
rebirth and a new history. Sadie trepans Perowne, boring a
hole in his brain to relieve the cranial pressure and to let
light in. Here, Williams differentiates between desire and
hope. As H. A. Williams says, "Hope is hope for we know
not what. . . . Desire, on the other hand, takes its form and
outline from what we already are."

All television can do is satisfy desire. *AC/DC,* with an un-
witting Christian impulse, is dramatizing hope as H. A.
Williams described it: "The prospect of the radically
new." [23] Perowne's trepanning is a kind of resurrection,
where the ultimate spiritual connection is made.

Perowne, in Sadie's words, is "out of names and games."

The stage directions indicate this transcendence: *"All cognitive clues to their behavior beginning to implode. . . .* Perowne *makes a series of minimal facial expressions, corresponding to no known emotion."* While Sadie chants in the background, "PLAY IT . . . PLAY IT . . . RELAY IT . . . RELAY it . . ." the last words are Perowne's revelation. Screaming and then smiling, he speaks in primal sounds, rendered on the printed page as hieroglyphics. In this moment, protean diffusion is resolved, and *AC/DC* fulfills the visionary intentions of Artaud. "The true purpose of theater is to create Myths. To express life in its immense universal aspect, and from that life to extract images in which we find pleasure in discovering ourselves." [24]

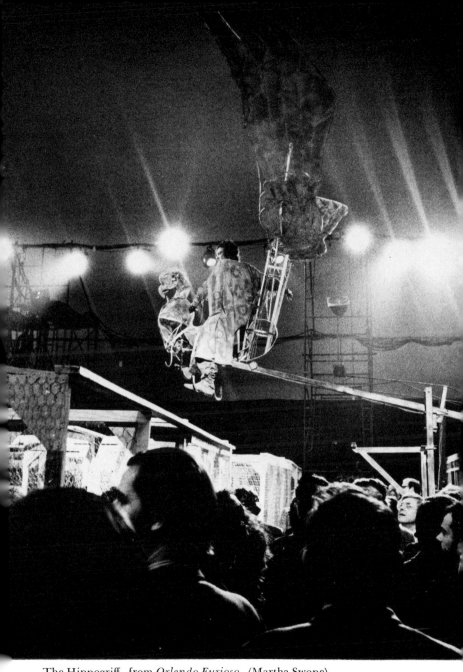

The Hippogriff—from *Orlando Furioso*. (Martha Swope)

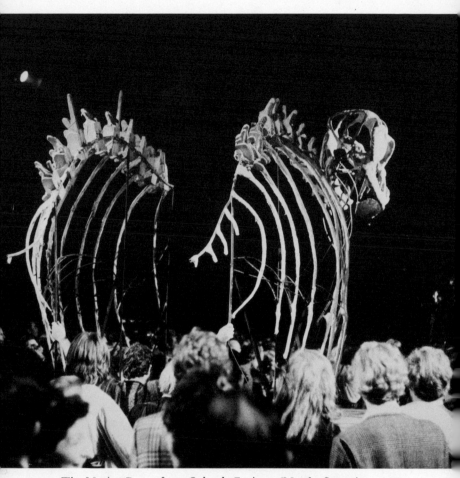

The Marine Bear —from *Orlando Furioso*. (Martha Swope)

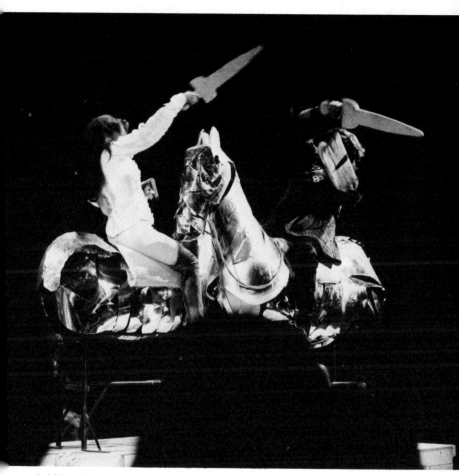

Soldiers fighting—from *Orlando Furioso*. (Martha Swope)

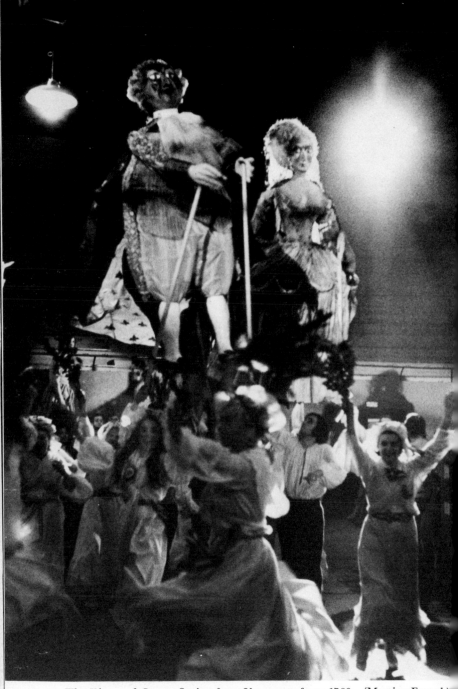

The King and Queen fleeing from Varennes—from *1789*. (Martine Franck)

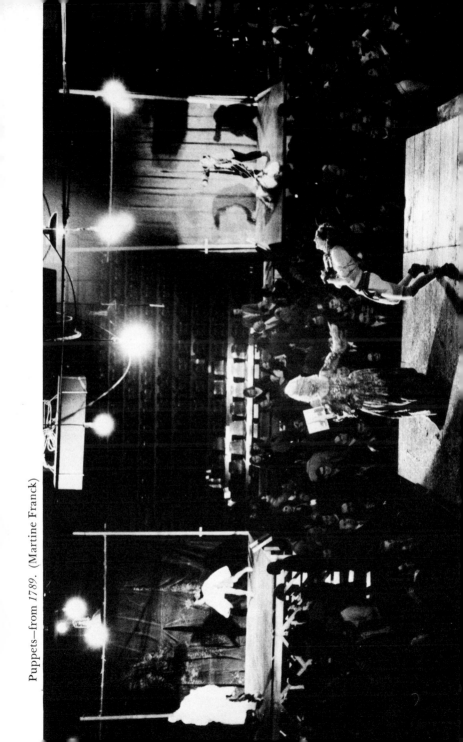

Puppets—from *1789*. (Martine Franck)

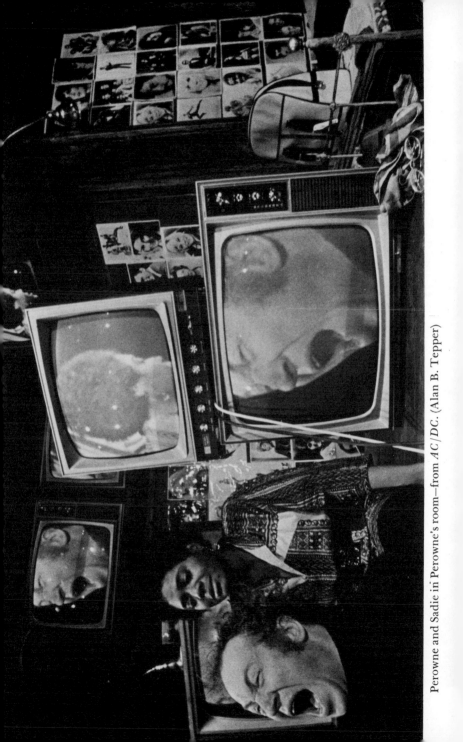

Perowne and Sadie in Perowne's room—from *AC/DC*. (Alan B. Tepper)

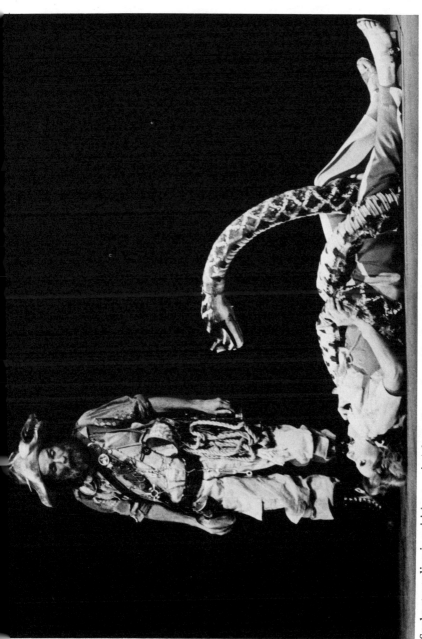

Snake strangling inquisitive tourist—from *Operation Sidewinder*. (Martha Swope)

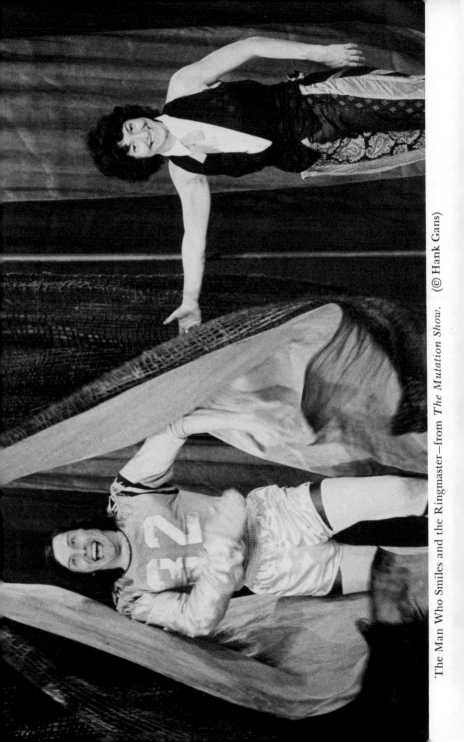

The Man Who Smiles and the Ringmaster—from *The Mutation Show*. (© Hank Gans)

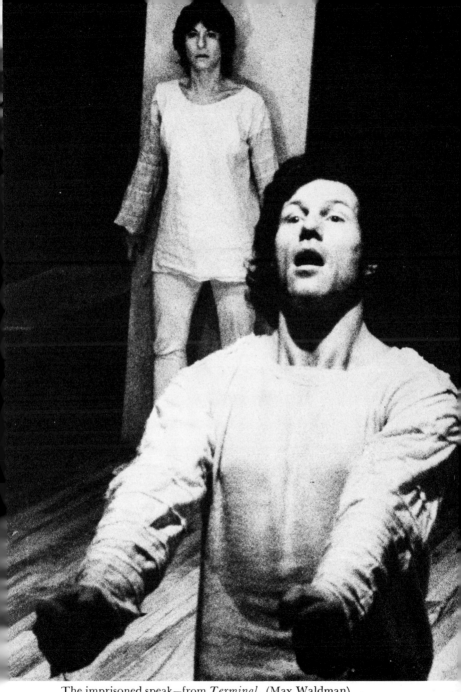

The imprisoned speak—from *Terminal*. (Max Waldman)

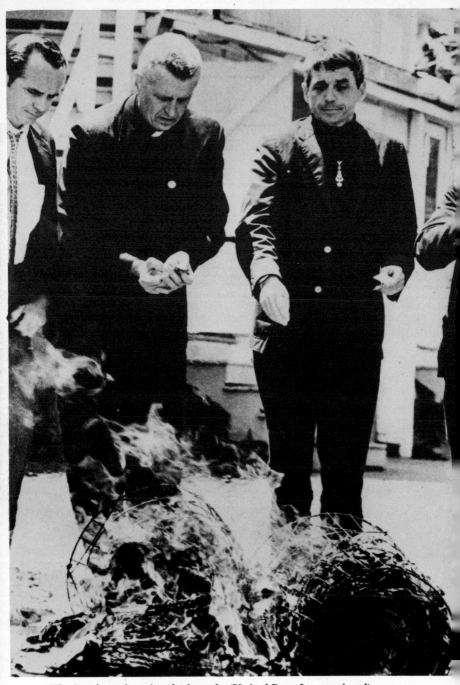

The Berrigans burning draft cards. (United Press International)

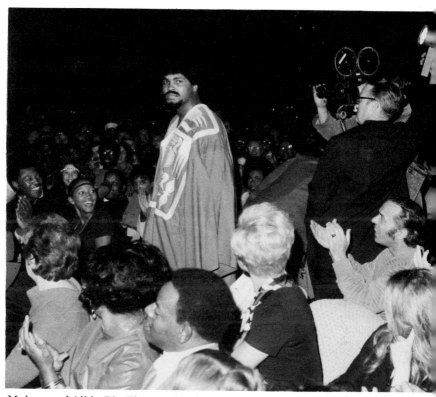

Muhammad Ali in *Big Time Buck White*. (Wide World)

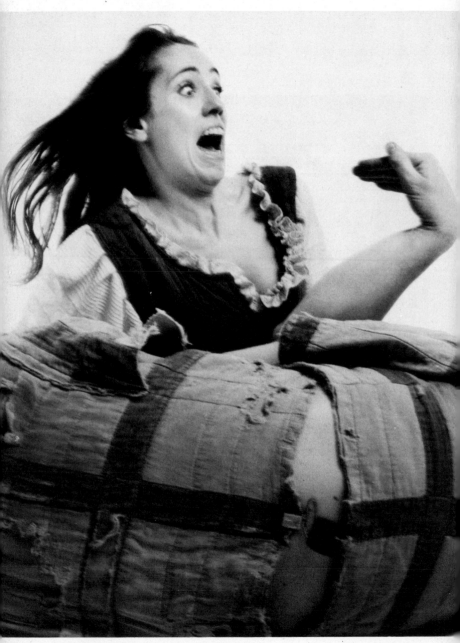

Alice and the Sea Serpent—from *Alice in Wonderland*. (Richard Avedon)

PERFORMANCES

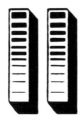

The Berrigans

Satyagraha [non-violent resistance] is a
process of educating public opinion such that
it covers all elements of the society and in the
end makes itself irresistible.

—GANDHI

Saints have always made a spectacle of their faith. They are
signs: turning their inner convictions of purity and love into
public events. In the highest sense of the word, they are actors, and they teach by making scenes. These acts not only
confirm but expand their faith. They are graphic demonstrations, vivid images which transcend barriers of knowledge and speak to the heart. Saint Francis of Assisi believed
"all brothers ought to preach by their actions." His costume
dramatized the humility and simplicity of the Christian
faith; his dedication to a life of poverty and service was its
living example. His public acts communicated directly to
the people. The Berrigans and the other seven Catholics,

who burned draft files with a crude napalm solution and who are now the Catonsville Nine, must be considered in this tradition: prophetic actors, celebrating the life of the spirit by exhibiting their willingness to die rather than contribute to the cruel, silent violence which is destroying America. Whether pouring blood into draft files or burning them, their intention is scenic. Spirit is cast against matter, nonviolence against violence. Having made their actions public, there is nothing the government can do to eradicate the omnipresence of their moral force. Every trumped-up charge, every jailing, expands the appeal and truth of their image. Their spiritual scenes become more vivid. Truth cannot be locked up or bombed away. It is irresistible.

The Berrigans understand the force of their public images. They dramatize a spiritual revolution, and theirs is not a revolution for the hell of it. Their actions are potent because they grow out of love, not hate; out of an acceptance of death, not a fear of it; out of fervent conviction, not flip nihilism. The simplicity of their performance provides a setting where the social sickness can be seen. Their symbolic and carefully controlled acts answer Dan Berrigan's question: "How do we help Americans get born, get going, get growing, get moving in a direction of recovery, recovery of what the Greeks would call the true way?" Inundated with a confusing mosaic of half-truths and censored images, we can only be renewed by images of exemplary action. These acts speak to the population the way Saint Francis taught the faith to the illiterate, fearful masses of the Middle Ages. The Catonsville Nine demonstrate rather than discuss. Argument is useless; words have become tools of betrayal. We know the facts of our war—the number killed, the cost, the acres destroyed, the amount of weaponry, the massacres—

but our knowledge does not stop the war. Facts and figures have no physical, tactile, moral outrage. In a "fantasy" war being fought in a "fantasy" land far from home, it is easy to forget. The lie of the society must be seen; the truth of renewal and the strangulation of America's moral confusion must be shown. Just as the Catonsville Nine are filled with a sense of the living presence of God, they themselves become a moral presence that facts and figures cannot deny. Once the purity of their performance is felt, the direction of history and of each individual life's role in it must be considered. The observer must make real emotional choices. As Philip Berrigan has written in *Prison Journals of a Revolutionary Priest*, "These are not times for building justice; these are times for confronting injustice. This we feel is the number one item of national business—to confront the entrenched, massive, complex injustice of our country. And to confront it justly, non-violently, and with maximum exposure of oneself and one's future."

The Trial of the Catonsville Nine, written by Daniel Berrigan, S. J., is an extension of the saintly compulsion to "make a scene." Like the actions of the group, it is a symbol and a sermon, a celebration and a sacrifice. Most of the real actors are in jail or underground, a retaliation typical of American society which trains its children from birth not to "act-up" or "make a scene" because it shames the community of the family. Those who take the roles of the Catonsville Nine, recounting the origins of their disenchantment with U.S. foreign policy and bearing witness to their moral concern, become disciples, doing the Nine's work in the world. This is a passion play: a testament of faith. It is not asking for pity, just for the privilege of displaying its commitment. The only gauge by which it can be judged is the clarity and joyous resignation by which it defines and communicates the spirituality of the group. On stage, the trial debate which was hidden from public scrutiny by the mass media is made visible; the story is extended beyond the indelible image of nine well-dressed, polite men and women bowing their heads in prayer while draft files burn in front of them. It is no coincidence that the play does not end with Berrigan's testament of sacrifice after the court sentence, "We agree this is the greatest day of our lives." Instead, as the lights fade out on the stage, their symbolic act is reborn on film. This is the source of their legitimacy, the primal exhibition of their moral courage. The Berrigans and their scenes are not only compelling, but necessary.

The life-love of the Catonsville Nine is too profound, the consequences of their actions too important to applaud. This is no sentimental journey. Their actions have consequences in our lives: they haunt the soul. Silently, in awe, and in astonished recognition of their righteousness, we file out of the church. This is the heady mixture of joyful discovery and fearful responsibility Saint Francis aroused in the crowds who followed him. "For what else are the servants of God," he wrote, "than his singers, whose duty is to lift up the hearts of men and move them to spiritual joy." Saint Francis dramatized faith through struggle; so do the Catonsville Nine. In our frantic materialism, we have forgotten the inner calm of the just, the potency and nobility of the truly spiritual act. No wonder the government is so afraid of the Berrigans; truth is the most subversive weapon of all.

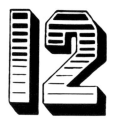

Open Theatre's *Terminal*

Tear-gas canisters blazed like falling stars as they streaked into the Cambridge side street, popping into noxious clouds of blue-gray smoke. Choking, crying, scattering like skittish zebras at the sight of jackals, the Harvard students leaped over their dormitory walls and rushed for safety. The gas was everywhere: even in their rooms. In the street, the helmeted task force marched, like brutal conquistadores, impervious and undaunted by a powerless enemy. When they retreated, the students rushed back into the night after them: taunting, throwing bricks at colleges and stores, starting fires, looting shops for the thrill of a free pair of bell-bottoms. Standing on a wall, watching the spectacle, I thought of the Open Theatre's *Terminal.* "We come among the living to call upon the dead. There are bones beneath this house. . . ." The Open Theatre's haunting litany became clear in the face of the fatuous violence of the riot, which was a pageant of how deeply the society has been touched by death and how numb it is to life. Even the radicals who pelted police cars with bricks and punched out parking meters yelling, "The streets belong to the people," had lost a reverence for life in the process of petty rebellion.

To respect life, we must understand death—the precise boundaries of an ending. "This is your last chance to use your eyes. This is the last chance to use your voice. This is the last chance to use your legs." How difficult, yet how necessary, it was to suffer these words in *Terminal*, to force the mind to imagine what it most feared. Watching *Terminal*, I realized that theater itself is so often an escape from death. The conventional killings, the eloquent last words eliminate the grim immediacy and horror of an ending by fitting death within the comfortable machinery of melodrama. To confront death so brazenly in *Terminal* is to rediscover humility. There was nothing humble in the Cambridge streets where the display of dumb power and futile resistance were reminders of America's arrogant sense of immortality: a myth sustained on the right by technology and power, and on the left by drugs and the hope of revolution. In dramatizing death so clinically, the Open Theatre aspires to renew the audience's sense of life and the need for compassionate change.

A shot rang out. The student crowd stampeded again, their feet clattering like hoofs in a stone canyon. In panic, people separated from their companions and became confused. The noise reverberated like the staccato pounding with which the Open Theatre summon up the dead in their somber, ferocious ballet. They move in rigid, angular steps; they never touch one another. "Let them take my body. Let them use my tongue. Let the dead come through. And let it begin with me. . . ." *Terminal* guides an audience into a purgatory. The actors, in hospital dressing gowns as pale as shrouds, move in free-form, abstract patterns. The actors, like the rioters, become a shifting blur of sound and movement: frightened then bold, furious then playful. Voices scream a wordless testament. Shami Chaikin, pinioned to a large wooden bed as she tips sideways (but never forward) with her burden. In Cambridge, the frolic passing for ferment bore out her moment of frustration and stasis.

The Harvard riot was made in the name of the dead and the dying: those who die in Vietnam and in the ghettos and in the schools. I wanted to embrace their anger; but, in the rioters, I saw ghosts of revolutionaries seeking not responsibility but revenge. In the fumes, they looked like specters. I remembered Peter Maloney's owlish eyes in *Terminal*: a walking skeleton. His song, methodical and military, counterpointed an infernal jig in which the dancer spun out a tale of despair, "And my people live like slaves." Maloney, saluting, chanted, "Yes, sir. Said Yes when I wanted to say No. And dead because I said Yes. And dead because you said Yes. Dead before and dead again because I never knew what the FUCK I was saying Yes to!"

We have contributed to the death of others and yearn to purify ourselves. The paradox is this: in the process of saying No, do we cherish life? In *Terminal*, the dying imagined their Final Judgment, slinking in a circle on their bellies while the Archangel reads the judgments through a bullhorn. The words indict our mediocrity and underscore the living death which passes for a way of life. "The Judgment of your life is your life. You neither faced your death nor participated in your life. But straddled the line between one place and another longing for both." In the riot, there was only a sense of bravado and heady heroic mission. Students brought down wastepaper baskets full of water so the gassed could clear their eyes; Weathermen directed traffic and snarled at defiant cars, "This is liberated territory." But in this climate, there was no freedom. In the excitement, that joyousness of would-be combat, there was little humility and less love.

Events happened too fast for action to be infused with a careful sense of morality. The street was noisy; the night was wild and frantic. The imagination fed off this surface excitement; whereas *Terminal* revived the memory of stillness from which language and movement first emerged and to which they will return. The rioters were prankish, never confronting death. The actors held the experience in front of their audiences, making them watch their own evasions. *Terminal* forced choices. "You saw. You saw. You can't say you didn't." The lines echo through the event. The words are a challenge and an indictment. By re-creating the agonizing simplicity of man's final moments and the hypocrisy of his embalming, *Terminal* sends the audience away with a passion for preserving the gift of life: its exciting variety, its possibilities, its essential sweetness. *Terminal* makes you conscious of death and the limits of time, so that you realize the necessity of taking your life into your own hands. But unlike the Harvard riot, the call to action is mixed with a compassion and commitment approaching love.

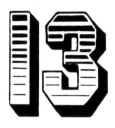

Open Theatre's *The Mutation Show*

We are all mutants—malleable protoplasm either pulverized into shape by the culture or pushing our way beyond it. The verbs for the modern experience are words of transformation. We are warped by the political betrayals, shrunken by the technological explosion, beaten by the system, eroded by the environment, expanded by drugs. We go through "changes" and glorify our "trips," but the journey is simply that of survival—*homo sapiens* groping for ways to adapt to alien territory. In this urgent and hysterical climate, modern man seems less a character and more a cartoon—flattened by the speed of living, simplified by the vectors of his greed and his despair.

On stage, only the grotesque can condense and evoke the combination of ugliness and exaggeration which is the urban American condition. The grotesque makes a myth of ugliness, distancing the pain while acknowledging the seriousness of the situation. The grotesque, wrote Northrop Frye, is "the comic imitation of tragedy." Where the Open

Theatre's *Terminal* faced the subject of death with a tragic earnestness, *The Mutation Show* is a liberation from that tone, unleashing a ghoulish carnival of life-forces at play in a suffocating universe. *The Mutation Show* is a capriccio of the social cancer; and, although it is a work-in-progress, it is already vivid, bold, and thrilling.

The grotesque combines irony with low comedy. From the first moment, when the Open Theatre's musician walks artlessly to the edge of the audience with a piece of paper in her hand, the Open Theatre is firmly in control of their brilliant theatrical intention. She reads a list of don'ts to the audience.

No smoking. . . .
No taking pictures. . . .

At these first deadpan words, the expectant audience feels its sense of excitement shrivel. Annoyed at the rigidity, the audience nonetheless is imaginatively prepared to accept any imposed pattern of response. The list continues.

No crinkling paper. . . .
Try to avoid having sexual fantasies about the people in the play. . . .
Try to avoid having sexual fantasies about the person to the right or left of you. . . .

The juxtaposition makes us laugh. The Open Theatre was just kidding. But, of course, it's not. For in that moment, we have experienced the first mutation, not on the stage but in ourselves. We accommodate ourselves to any set of rules. The audience has learned to adapt; it barely notices these little psychic adjustments which are all part of coping. *The Mutation Show* focuses on this sense of latent acquiescence and passivity.

The freaks' parade begins on the next beat, and as at a circus side show, we watch, astonished and relieved, that we are not like them, although in some ways we share their deformities. The Mutants are announced by the rhythmic grunts of The Ringmaster, who kicks and struts through her palsied dance dressed in a black vest and red string tie. Beginning in words and moving into pantomime, The Ringmaster becomes as brutal a gargoyle as those she introduces: The Bird Lady, The Man Who Smiles, The Man Who Hits Himself, The Thinker, The Petrified Man. They each make their entrances, with their own signatures of sound and gesture that are orchestrated through the piece as visual links between their transformations. Are they animals or human beings? This theatrical confusion is apt for the grotesque, where man and animal meet and merge in emotional exaggeration.

"The Boy in the Box," squawks the Ringmaster, pointing to a simple wooden box. "One day he was torn from his box and carried to a hill where he was left." An actor reaches in the box and tries to pull out the body by a leg. The box tumbles forward and the boy is visible. As in a breech delivery, he is cramped and tumbled upside down. His first contact with the world is by his feet. He stares at his toes. The Petrified Man's fear is in The Boy's soft, high-pitched sounds. He is carried up the hill on the back of his captor. In a brilliant piece of physical invention, The Boy and his captor mime their wonder and trepidation at what they see. They freeze at moments of insight. At one point The Boy is almost horizontal to the stage: the acrobatic feat never loses the sense of fascination and fear that keeps The Boy clinging to his captor's back. Gradually, as they near the summit, The Boy senses he will be abandoned. The Boy's arms wrap themselves like weeds around his captor's neck, only to be brushed aside. Finally, The Boy wrestles the captor to the ground but cannot hold him. The Boy is left alone, whimpering. The traumas of birth and separation are physicalized with exquisite precision.

The capture of The Animal Girl ("She was raised with animals. She ate and slept and drank with an animal pack. One day she was torn from her cave and carried away and made civilized") is, in this allegory, the fettering of spontaneity. Gasping, crawling, frantic, The Animal Girl is decoyed into a lasso which is pulled tight. Her strangulation and pain are accompanied by the howling of her pack and by the chant of her captors.

> We will name her.
> We will give her words.
> We will caress her.

Categories restrict; words betray; affection in the name of possession smothers. Later, The Animal Girl is lowered into shoes and taught to walk, first in flats and then more boldly in the unnatural steps of high heels. Like The Animal Girl, we assume the postures of our captors. As *The Mutation Show* implies, being caught in someone else's dream can be seductive fun but also soul-destroying.

Like the circus, *The Mutation Show* turns violence into laughs. The Ringmaster is banged on the head with a paper hoop that rips apart. Eggs are smashed. Instruments are pounded and battered with an anarchic, brutal cacophony. The Man Who Hits Himself smashes from inside the box, and finally breaks out. His body is bloodied. He can hardly see. Change always takes its toll. The culture is cluttered with the debris of blown minds, aiming for some bypass circuit of the society—amnesiacs, dropouts, revolutionaries crippled by a frustrated dream of breaking through. The Man Who Hits Himself evokes all this as he scans the new world. He talks of light, the intimation of some higher spiritual order. Bludgeoned and numbed, he cannot pursue it.

> Nothing with me in my box all the time closed by the box I was alone with only my fluids came out of here and here and here and here and then suddenly out of the box I saw for the first time only that one time saw light, light, light, behind my eyes. . . . And then I saw . . . many boxes with holes and people going out of the boxes and people going in and out of the boxes made a noise. And the noise was in my head. . . . I don't know if this happened to me or to someone else. But I know it happened.

Not all mutations are negative. For one scene, the performing artifice is dropped. The actors stand behind enlarged snapshots of themselves in their youth. The musician announces their histories. The pictures do not show the mutated faces of the actors. Now, their faces are deepened, lined, articulate because of the energy they have learned to focus in their bodies. One of the actors, Ray Barry, was a gardener, a construction worker, an English teacher, a sculptor. Another, Paul Zimet, won the American Legion Citizenship Award in the sixth grade. The pictures—like Shami Chaikin's Debbie Reynolds' pose complete with kerchief around her neck—have no sense of excess; they are devoid of any intimation of spiritual struggle. These performers who have discovered the grotesque in life and in themselves had, as adolescents, no intuition of this in front of the cameras. Playing has kept the actors open, even their theater takes its name from this affinity with growth, this aspiration for a divine milieu.

At the finale, The Mutants make a concert of their sounds—panting, running in place, hushing, rustling. In this panorama of limitation, words spring out of the tapestry of vocal patterns. The Mutants posture, but do not discover. "This is not my real voice," says The Thinking Lady, practicing the word "this" at various pitches. The Petrified Man adjusts his poses to the tone of his voice, a sense of confusion behind his apparent control.

> I speak it the way I hear it.
> I do it the way I was taught it.
> I see it the way it was shown to me.
>
> Why did they teach me to speak this way
>   if I was not meant to be a clergyman?

He lapses into a civilized stance. Even for the clergy, the route to a transcendent experience is blocked.

The Mutants twitch and grimace. Physically stalemated, some stand, others sit. Their heads nod, their bodies heave with the quiet music of breathing. At the end as in the beginning, the Mutants are trying to find the right words, trying to find the right voice. The Open Theatre imbues these actions with a spiritual intensity. From them, we learn and understand that fantasy is "instant mutation"; a new source of energy and the beginning of a higher understanding.

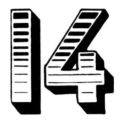

Ike and Tina Turner

The salmon in me is going upstream.

She says, "We don't do nothin' nice 'n' easy; we do things nice 'n' rough." This time I'm ready. I can handle it. My hands are pressed tight against the brass rail, my feet are firmly planted on the carpet. I'm Standing Room Only at Carnegie Hall, and Tina Turner is talking to me. I've got her clearly focused in my binoculars. Her nipples loom like the muddy craters of the Sea of Tranquillity beneath the purple net of her dress. (How did she know purple was my color?) Her nails are sharp and buffed to a menacing shine. Her hair lashes across her face. Her knees scrape the stem of the microphone. She says, "What you hear is what you get!" Tina is voracious. She knows her hunger and ours. I have to put my binoculars down. There's so much to get, and so little time.

"Hi, everybody!"

"Hi, Tina!" we say, forgetting where we are. We know Annie Mae Bullock's stage name now. She likes to hear us say it again and again. She is toying with us; but that's why we came—to be played with. She is visible, and with a vengeance. She has said good-by to bad times. In every combustible gyration and ecstatic shuffle of her performance, she puts mileage between the past and her gaudier present. She stops time, and she knows it. Tina's presence is her power. She lifts grown men out of their seats; they wave at the stage; they talk to it. She lures them out of themselves in an elaborate contest of wills. She knows she has energy, and every performance is a conquest which not only renews us but makes her stronger. She competes with the electronic guitar, played by Ike, backing her up. (She *can* make a deeper, purer sound.) She tests the resilience and prowess of the Ikettes who dance with her. (She *does* move faster.) She comes up against the audience with a street-fighter's lust for battle. And she wins. (We want her to conquer us.) And wins completely. She surrounds us with her sound and her excess. She is outrageous, and this is her glory. People are coaxed out of isolation and into a community.

> I wanna take you Higher,
> Higher,
> Higher,
> Higher. . . .

With each bellow, she fans the passion of the audience. This is total emotional catharsis. Carnegie Hall is not Freak City, and yet people are standing on their seats, moving down the aisles just to be near her. She has enough life for a whole auditorium; people move toward this luminous presence like moths to a light. Her energy is superhuman. The audience is *feeling* something. They are grateful and awed.

Everything about Tina's act creates the illusion of mythic gesture. When she backsteps into the chorus line, the theatrical effect is thrilling. Who is she? Part animal, part wonder-woman. She swims. She bucks. She scoops her arms in the air like a cowboy cracking a bullwhip. She teases an audience with the innuendo of her voice. She can make them remember their sex; and her body—as sleek and playful as a pony—is also a metaphor which inspires an elaborate reverie. The magic has to be faced, not magnified. On stage, she is larger than life. Television shrinks her; films miss the riveting, erotic immediacy of her performance. Even my binoculars are unfair for this kind of spectator sport. The illusion is perfectly calibrated for the naked eye. If you look too closely, the hand-movements become isolated "tricks"; the "steps" seem like simple, rudimentary prancing which somehow passes for choreography. And so you put away all the accessories. Quickly. The need for the illusion is too great; the longing for Tina's artifice to seize you, absorb you into the kinetic whirlwind on stage is too necessary. No part of the stage is silent or immobile. Every moment is filled with the friction of movement and change.

"Now I'm gonna be serious," Tina says. "I'm gonna sing this one for the men." I know there are words to the song. Tina is whispering, "I want you to give it to me. . . ." And Ike is replying, "Ooh, shit baby. . . ." But I'm captivated by the drama underneath the words. I know the Ikettes are bopping dumbly in the darkness behind her, the fringe of their white dresses floating like seaweed. But all I can hear is the rasping gurgle in Tina's voice. The purple pin-spot focuses on her. It's hard to see. She's almost invisible, except for her hands. Tina runs the flat of her palm along the microphone. She takes both hands and, slowly, without touching the mechanism, works her way up. (Can't we keep this to ourselves, Tina? Does it have to be out here with everybody watching?)

"Don't choke on it," somebody yells. Nobody laughs. Tina is walking in their dreams, too.

And at the finale, with the strobe lights flashing, Tina churning in her familiar gyrations, the audience clapping and stomping, a cloud of smoke suddenly billows up from the floor. From the loud speaker, we hear a voice blaring

TINA TURNER
TINA TURNER
TINA TURNER
TINA TURNER
TINA TURNER
TINA TURNER

When the haze rises, Tina has disappeared. Vanished. The effect is perfect. There are no curtain calls, nothing except the program to remind us that Tina has been among us. This is as it should be. We care about Tina with a spiritual concern. Like all religious figures, Tina is both visible and invisible. Whoever created her act knows how to make a myth and keep it vibrant.

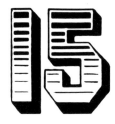

Maurice Chevalier

The headline is: "M. Chevalier: Comedian Popular for His Warmth and Gaiety."

It hurts to see the words: their icy matter-of-factness remind me how intimate Chevalier had become, how rare and enduring the bond of his performances. I never met him. I saw his song and dance only occasionally. But like every master of intimacy, one night in his company could sustain a lifetime's affection. Chevalier and I were friends: the way all living legends find their way into our dream landscape. I needed him not for what he said, but for the effect he had on audiences, on me. He could bring people together; he could coax them out of their numbness and locate for them new resources of feeling. He made us momentarily unafraid of our failures; and we owed him a debt greater than applause. He received—like any star of his magnitude—our care with humility and grace. I needed him. He needed me. It was our silent understanding: the same he had with each and every person who was touched by his brand of Gallic blarney.

Mistinguett, who danced Chevalier to fame in the *Folies-Bergère* (1910), declined to explain Chevalier's particular hypnotic effect on the world. *"Il a le fluide,"* she said. *Le fluide* is a code word for the mercurial genius of a star turn, the capacity to remain continually fresh and surprising and true. It is a gift, a hunger, a chemistry which allows a performer through the metaphor of his gestures and voice to show himself to the public and to confirm, in that risk, an invisible need in the mass consciousness. Being the son of a man who was a theatrical legend, I find this terrain eerie and evocative. And as I grow older, I think I understand more clearly the responsibility and mystery of legendary figures.

A legend knows his power, but not its source. He never questions the mystery of his gift, or fully understands the impact and meaning to an audience. He is the Rorschach blot of his time. The public interprets him to fulfill their own needs. His technique and performance refine—to a kind of purity—his skill at being himself. This is an intuitive process; for when a performer, like Charlie Chaplin, understands his intellectual meaning to an audience, his art suffers.

True genius carries with it a gentleness and openness that comes with an enduring sense of wonder and surprise at the luck of talent. Egotism, or in Chevalier's case, bonhomie, may hide this awe. Yet if legendary performers do not know why they have been blessed, they know how to protect their power. Silence is crucial to legend. A star, like an angel, must have the ability to be present and to vanish. The great stars are hermits at heart: criticism cannot pluck out the core of their mystery; the media cannot flush them out into the open of late-night talk shows. Their true life and only statement is in performance. They are artificers; and no magician tells his tricks. Intuitively, they know that their excitement and lasting appeal is in their energy on stage, not what's behind the scenes. In his last year, Chevalier secluded himself and his anguish from even his closest friends. He lived alone at his country estate. He prayed in his garden. Only his immediate family and staff were allowed to see his body. This was his wish; and his instinct was in keeping with the demands of his legend. As a dream figure, the public must not remember him as immobile, static, decrepit. His immortality is in the resilient memory of his movement: the pouting lower lip, the naughty wink of his bedroom eyes, the straw hat dipping rakishly down over his forehead.

Legends are a bridge between generations: a valid currency of exchange when the coin of manners and morals has been devalued. Through film, the young—like their parents—grow up with the shared imagery of Groucho, W. C. Fields, Bogie, and hundreds of lesser lights. Yet as we move toward death, the celluloid legends remain miraculously in their prime. And the audience—having brought the legendary figure to life through its faith in him—also shares vicariously in the star's immortality: the reward of any true believer. The legends belong to us, and our possessiveness is visible in how we worship "their memory" by which we mean our memory of them; how we tear at their clothes, preserve their signatures, try to invade their privacy.

There is a special sadness when a stage legend passes away. The stage performer who has grown old with his audiences and still cavorts in front of them, leaves only memories of moments. He trades in transience. His gift is in stopping time and transforming it. In life, he is one of society's gaudiest victors; in death, one of its saddest specimens. Now, no stage performer can be assured of a lifetime in the theater. All the major theatrical legends have made movies, but few of the movies capture the soul and spellbinding excitement of the stage performance. Chevalier on film is a shadow of the man in person; Dietrich on the screen is a miniature compared to the seismic impact she has on stage. The same is true of clowns. Film could never capture the dangerous mayhem of Bobby Clark or Bert Lahr (except significantly when his energy was not in human but animal form as the Cowardly Lion).

Legends not only mold a sense of style and help us redefine our emotional mythology; they can lead us further into examining ourselves. What is gained by witnessing a stage performance is the quality of emotion and involvement. In front of us, the performing legends speak their own private language. Silence surrounds them. We ask nothing more than to be in their presence, to be warmed by their energy and their unique insight into experience. They have suffered and they have felt; and if their greatness is genuine and not synthetic, we do not lose ourselves, but recover fragments of our humanity.

And when one of the exemplary performers dies, he is profoundly to be mourned.

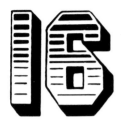

E. Y. Harburg

America is the only society which defines itself by a dream, not a reality. With his lyrics, E. Y. Harburg has given body and weight to his vision of social harmony, equality, and human resilience. Mr. Harburg calls himself a "minstrel"; but he knows that the lyric is a potent political tool. ("A song makes you feel a thought: a new idea can find a soft spot under a hard-hat.") No lyricist of the theater's older generation has been more inventive with the rhymed word or more deeply involved with the destiny of the nation. His wry questioning and painfully personal statements have a "re-evolutionary" potential. They are in our dreams. Harburg's songs have never let the society forget itself, reminding us of our small place on this galaxy, the simplicity of our needs and ideals, and how they have been betrayed: "Brother Can You Spare a Dime," "Over the Rainbow," "It's Only a Paper Moon," "Great Come-and-Get-It Day."

"I grew up when America had a dream and its people a hope," Harburg says. "The hope was there. The songs evolved with the sweetness of hope. . . . During that time, the middle classes were enjoying a partial paradise." In Harburg's most scathing indictments of the society, his songs still hold out the sense of benevolence in their playfulness. From *Finian's Rainbow* (1947), "Necessity" raises the question of poverty and the frustration that leads to crime.

> What is the curse,
> That makes the universe
> So all-bewilderin'.
>
> What is the hoax
> That just provokes
> The folks
> They call God's childerin.
>
> Necessity, necessity
> That most unnecessary thing, necessity!
> What throws the monkey wrench in
> A fellow's good intention?
> That nasty old invention,
> Necessity.

In his seventies, Mr. Harburg is talking the language of today's rebellion. He bridges generations; he is at the center of the nation's emotional history. He is asking for a decent society; an ethic of abundance, not scarcity. The delight of his lyrics is in their exuberant attack on difficult subjects with humor and intelligence. The lesson is the discovery of complex concepts—like the paradox of social mobility and class responsibility in America—put with such economy and verve, as "When the Idle Poor Become the Idle Rich" from *Finian's Rainbow*.

When the idle poor become the idle rich
You'll never know just who is who
Or who is which.
No one will see
The Irish or the Slav in you,
For when you're on Park Avenue,
Cornelius and Mike
Look alike.

On the Broadway treadmill, Mr. Harburg is the only lyricist to get genuinely comic with the cosmic. His very presence is an act of renewal; he is, to borrow F. R. Leavis's
concept, on "the line of wit" which leads from him to Bob
Dylan and the Beatles. Because Harburg takes the long-
view of society ("I look upon myself as a lyrical historian,
these are rhymed chronicles of the world"), he uses his satire to deflate ego. He doesn't need hashish, only history, to
put life into perspective. From his calypso musical *Jamaica*
(1957), the song "Napoleon" makes its wise and hilarious
point.

Napoleon's a pastry
Bismarck's a herring
Alexander's just a crème de cacao mixed with rum
And Hoo-oo-oover is a vacu-u-um.

Columbus is a circle—and a day-off.
Pershing is a square—what a pay off.
As for Caesar, he's just a salad on a shelf.
So, little brother, get wise to yourself.

Harburg's focus is not on glorifying the metropolis (Ira

Gershwin) or the contemporary (DeSylva, Brown, and Henderson) or romantic wistfulness (Larry Hart, Oscar Hammerstein). His songs, at their best, always come back to the question of spiritual and social survival. This gives them their lasting sinew. "Leave de Atom Alone" from *Jamaica* is indicative of how Harburg's concern and comic flair intermingle. Man's fatuity works its way into every rhyme. The word "atom" and "Adam" have a delicious, scary ambiguity here.

> Ever since de apple in the Garden of Eve,
> Man always fooling wid things that cause
>   him to grieve. . . .
> But not since de doomsday in old Babylon
> Did he fool wid anything so diabolical as the cyclotron.
> So, if you wish to avoid de most uncomfortable
>   trip to Paradise,
> You will be scientific and take my advice—
>
> Leave de atom alone.
> Leave de atom alone.
> Don't get smart alecksy
> Wid de galaxy.
> Leave atom alone. . . .

The humility which goes into the humor, the playfulness and the message of Harburg's songs, evolve from his sense of the human condition. The life cycle, in all its sadness, and glory, is worth singing about. Harburg was posing the predicament long before Robert Ardrey, Desmond Morris, and Konrad Lorenz had made the public conscious of itself as a species.

> Man, he eat the barracuda.
> Barracuda eat the bass,

Bass he eat the little flounder,
'Cause the flounder lower class.
Little flounder eat the sardine,
That's nature's plan.
Sardine eat little worm
Little worm eat man.

Harburg is an acrobat with words. He can juggle the English language into breathtaking convolutions—a game of intricacy and enlightenment, where the interior rhymes never lose the idea behind the song, but expand it. For instance, in *Finian's Rainbow*, a leprechaun who finds himself feeling human lust, sings:

Ev'ry *femme* that flutters by me
Is a flame that must be fanned;
When I can't fondle the hand I'm fond of
I fondle the hand at hand.

Harburg is himself a theatrical event. Within his small, puckish frame is a life with all the sadness and joy made visible. No contemporary lyricist can claim his scope. Harburg's love songs ("Last Night When We Were Young," "It's Only a Paper Moon," "Old Devil Moon," "Down with Love," "Happiness Is a Thing Called Joe") are in a class with the very best; but Harburg has also managed to turn his talents to serve Groucho Marx ("Lydia, the Tattooed Lady") and Bert Lahr ("Song of the Woodsman"). The parody, the political satire, the serious emotion, and the despair which come through all these oblique lyric tactics give Harburg's *œuvre* its exceptional quality.

"If I were born today, I don't think I could dissent with

humor and satire." This is precisely why Harburg is important. He fuses his lyrics—even in dissent—with a wonder and an infectious love of life. He is from a generation of older radicals from whom the young can learn both a respect for the living and a way of seeing beyond the apocalypse. "I Don't Think I'll End It All Today" from *Jamaica* turns to nature and humanity with all the contemporary *brio* of Ray Mungo discovering the Total Loss Farm.

> When I see de world and its wonders
> What is there to say?
> I don't think, oh, no, I don't think
> I'll end it all today.
> Fish in sea and sun in de heaven
> Sailboat in de bay . . .
> I don't think, oh, no, I don't think
> I'll end it all today.
>
> So many sweet things still on my list,
> So many sweet lips still to be kissed,
> So many sweet dreams still to unfold,
> So many sweet lies still to be told.

Rarely is our theater so rich in thought, emotion, and consciousness of craft. Harburg gives pleasure. His songs turn an audience back into itself. With him, an audience rediscovers emotions, memories, and ideas which confront our future as well as recall our past.

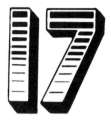

Comden and Green

To hear Betty Comden and Adolph Green tell it, the lyric is not coaxed into the world by applying the seat of the pants to the seat of the chair, but yanked from the imagination in a tornado of good spirits. After seeing them perform their work, it is hard to conceive of any song being written sitting down.

In their generosity, excitement, and enduring good will, Comden and Green incarnate the best of what is left of the Broadway myth. They themselves are myth-makers, creating an image of their world so gaudy and mysterious that one is dazzled by the surface and unquestioning of what lies beneath. They are jazzy, stylish,, up-to-the-minute pranksters, who have glided through this universe of pain with puckish insouciance. They have been rewarded for their carefree enthusiasm, and no wrinkle in their wardrobe or words from their mouths tell us that life is hard, cruel, indifferent, and mean. This is Broadway talking. They won't be serious: not about life or their considerable theatrical accomplishment. Although they never get down to details in a lecture, they leave an audience imagining that their lyrics are conceived something like this: Comden, svelte and shrewd, stands by the window. Green, with the protruding chin and elevated lower lip of a sunfish, is humming a snatch of the tune in the vicinity of the piano. They both get the same brilliant idea. Comden gives the first word, Green the second. They go back and forth, matching each other word for word in a contest of fancy. The pace quickens. Green caroms around the room—pirouetting, doing double takes, flinging Comden around the study like an Apache dancer. Sometimes he forgets Comden and just bounces off the wall. They have a song! They go to the phone. They call Lenny Bernstein. They sing it to him. He loves it. They're a hit!

Comden and Green "sell" their songs. They are performers—having written themselves into their first Broadway musical, *On the Town* (1944)—and they want their songs to be their surrogates on stage: dazzling spectators with energy and festival spirits. For them, the lyric is first and foremost a vehicle of fun; and then, surrender. The lyric is a means of touching the heart and evoking instant response—the shock of delight, the immediate adulation are the ingredients which, in its heyday, turned Broadway theaters into temples, its artists into secular saints. Comden and Green could sing the telephone book (they match the words of the "Marseillaise" to the tune of "Take Me Out to the Ball Game") and make it *opéra bouffe*. In this, they are truly American—giving us a sense of succeeding without the real experience of struggle.

As a team, their strength (and final limitation) is knowing how to please and doing it with ease. Their songs rarely show us depth; but, at their best, they exhibit the literacy and the voluptuous devotion to living the good life which— like it or not—is at the center of the American experience. Their songs of optimism have a conviction and excitement which touch something real at the core of their personalities and substitute for a philosophy. From *Subways Are for Sleeping* (1961):

> Take each day
> And gather the rosebuds in it.
> Live each minute. . . .
> Everyday that comes
> Comes once in a lifetime. . . .
> Think of now.
> Tomorrow is waiting in the wings.
> Who knows what it brings?
> While the future waits,
> The present swings. . . .

Comden and Green glory in the moment. They seize it, like they take the stage, with a voracious appetite. In the days of the revue, their wit, their brassy facility, could be punctuated with the black-out. Their knowledge of music, their love of the cultural figures in New York filters through their songs as happily as in life. In *Two on the Aisle* (1951), they wrote a first-act finale, for Dolores Gray and Bert Lahr, which could be considered a definitive, boffo Broadway epiphany. "Catch Our Act at the Met" gives Comden and Green a chance to sharpen their satire; season the fun with a sprinkling of classical allusions and blend it into a frothy, upbeat Broadway caprice.

LAHR and GRAY: Yes sirree, feelin' grand
We're an act that's in demand.
Yea, we're workin' steady
We're all set.
Got ourselves a season at the Met.
The opera once was a long-haired thing.
'Til they got a new manager, Rudolph Bing.

LAHR: And now the Met's gone vaudeville.
GRAY: He cleaned out the Horseshoe.
LAHR: Dusted off the pianahs.
GRAY: Dressed up the stage.
LAHR: And undressed the sopranahs

TOGETHER: Yeah, we don't need that Rodgers
    and Hammerstein
We're not dependent on the Theatre Guild
Cause you can always catch our act at the Met.
LAHR: I'll be Siegfried.
GRAY: And I'll be Brunhilde.
LAHR: De *Götterdämmerung*-a.
GRAY: De *Götterdämmerung*-a.

TOGETHER: . . . Italian opera, French and Dutch
Now have that added Broadway touch.
And look at what a smash they made of *Fledermaus*
Variety says: MOUSE PACKS HOUSE. . . .

This is what the trade calls a "show-stopper." The immediacy of its references, the fullness of the comic idea, the theatricality of its construction can paralyze an audience with delight. History may not remember the words; but the confidence in Comden and Green's tone, the sureness of the attack in the song are indicative of their musical and satiric talents working at their peak.

Comden and Green are not dreamers. They are city folks, who sing best about the sophistication and excitement of the metropolis ("New York, New York"). They are satisfied with the present; the lack of abrasion in their world does not breed that deep-seated longing that inspires dreams. They do not yearn for what lies over the rainbow; and, when called upon to write fantasy (as in their work for the famous Mary Martin *Peter Pan*), they can turn out polished, capable lyrics as sweet as they are uncommitted. Their idea of childhood has no real faith in dreaming, as vague in lyric form as it is in memory.

> I know a place where dreams are born
> And time is never planned.
> It's not in any chart
> You must find it in your heart:
> Never Never Land.

Comden and Green are best when writing the sharp, brittle, punchy lyrics of comedy. Rosalind Russell said to them before opening in *Wonderful Town* (1953), "I want something that goes 'Da-da-da-da-da-da, joke.'" That, they can deliver. For Miss Russell they invented the amusing "One Hundred Ways to Lose a Man":

> Throw your knowledge in his face,
> He'll never try for second base.

Their best score, *Bells Are Ringing* (1956), written for their good friend Judy Holliday, has a lyrical pathos which is it-

self an intuition of Miss Holliday's character. "Just in
Time" and "The Party's Over" are now standards from the
show, exhibiting that hint of loneliness which few of their
other show tunes pursue as ruthlessly. A great many of the
Comden and Green lyrics need to be performed for their
drama and sly humor to be experienced. "The Party's
Over" is in itself a dramatic monologue, where the lyrics
flow unobtrusively, at the same time pinpointing the world
of artifice and illusion (the exhaustion of the effort) which
these two myth-makers instinctively know.

> The party's over.
> It's time to call it a day.
> No matter how you pretend
> You knew it would end this way.
> It's time to wind up the masquerade,
> Just make your mind up
> The piper must be paid.

At their best, Comden and Green were *au courant,* but that
current has flowed by them. Still ebullient, still posh, still
high on their optimism—their lyric performance has a frantic gaiety which foreshadows the end of an era.

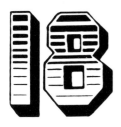

Lenny Bruce

In *Flying High* (1930), Bert Lahr simulated pissing in a bottle for a Broadway audience. The laugh was clocked at one minute and thirty seconds. "You can do almost anything on stage if you do it as if you haven't the slightest idea there's something wrong with what you're doing." All the great early comedians were rambunctious and vulgar; all shared Bert Lahr's belief that "dirty" was more in the style than in the content. There were ways of "getting around" a snappy story or "getting away" with a suggestive bit of business. They found them, and brought the animal instinct back into the paying customers' polite expectations of play. But truth, in their performances, evolved in spite of their passion to cater and to succeed within the system. Lenny Bruce is the only serious comic performer to emerge since the era of the great clowns, and the difference between the old and the new can be seen in the opening caper of one of Bruce's gritty *shticks:* "If you've ever seen this bit before, I'm going to piss on you." There was no innocence in Lenny Bruce's act, even if there was in his soul. Bad-mouth, manic Yiddish chatterbox, Lenny Bruce was always—by his own admission—"Hip." He was also direct—as direct as the law would let him be. He leveled the clown's anarchic spirit straight at the society. Bruce was among the first of many modern protesters to discover that slapstick had not died with burlesque but survived in the streets and in the law courts.

Both the source of Bruce's genius and his self-destruction stem from a martyr's fundamental simplicity. As with all great clowns, the image of saint and buffoon coalesce. Bruce's legendary obscenity case for which 3000 pages of testimony were compiled, on which one movie and now a Broadway play focus, was fought for a "crime" that carried a sentence of only between four to twelve months in jail. Clearly, the meaning of the trial was larger than the penalty. The same purity of motive forced him to ask basic questions, to go back to the roots of words and emotions, to explore what words and actions are in actuality and what they become in fantasy. ("To" is a preposition, "come" is a verb, etc.) His curiosity extended to his performance. On stage, he listened to himself and found himself discovering new areas of satire. He was vulnerable because his improvisations had access to his deepest, most troubling emotions; and he would not hide them, choosing to exhibit his despair through the mockery of laughter. The anger in his comedy evolved from this sense of profound betrayal: an almost childish faith in the purity of things. (He dedicates *How to Talk Dirty and Influence People* to "all true followers of Christ and his teachings; in particular to a true Christian—Jimmy Hoffa—because he hired ex-convicts as, I assume, Christ would have.") In many of Bruce's best routines, the springboard for his inventions came from specific definitions of words. "In the classic sense of the word" is a Brucism that recurs throughout his analysis of the society. One routine not included in the collage of his material incorporated by Julian Barry in *Lenny* stresses Bruce's semantic battle with the culture and also his ruthless naïveté: ideas which never find their way into his uptown sainthood.

> Sometimes I take poetic license with you, and you are offended. Now this is just with semantics—dirty words. Believe me, I am not profound. This is something I assume someone must have laid on me because I do not have an original thought. I am screwed. I speak English. That's it. I was not born in a vacuum. Every thought I have belongs to somebody else. I am not placating you by making the following statement: I want to help you with your dirty-word problem—there are none. And I'll spell it out logically for you.
>
> Here is a toilet. Specifically—that's all we're concerned with here, specifics—if I can tell you a dirty-toilet joke we must have a dirty toilet. That's what we're talking about—a toilet. If we take this toilet and boil it and it's clean, I can never tell you specifically a dirty toilet joke about this toilet. This toilet's a clean toilet now. Obscenity is a human manifestation. The toilet has no central nervous system, no level of consciousness. It is not aware. It is a dumb toilet. It cannot be obscene. It's impossible. If it could be obscene, it could be cranky. It could be a Communist toilet, a traitorous toilet. It can do none of these things. This is a dopey toilet, jim.

In his maturity, Bruce's routines blended with jazz and sometimes sounded like it—eccentric, extended riffs mixing mumbled asides with street talk and social observations. "Men are carnal, *definitely*. You put a guy in the Joint and he'll schtupp anything—mud." But whoever Bruce was, his myth overlooks roots he never forgot: his passion for tinsel town. Bruce was corny; nostalgic for *softig* chippies, flashy cars, the seedy bleakness of the nightclub circuit. Bruce exposed social taboos; but his hunger was palpable and more conventional. A large part of himself was trapped in the Grade-B movie of his mind.

In *Lenny*, the announcer says, "AND NOW, LENNY BRUCE. LADIES AND GENTLEMEN—LENNY BRUCE." There is a weird but real excitement. The old hint of danger feeds the applause. Cliff Gorman bounces on stage, grabs the mike, and starts the intimate conversation which leads to a fantasy of Father Flotsky. The audience howls; most of them have never heard this material before, and each line's surprise is worth its weight in gold. Gorman is an excellent performer; his body has a feline quickness; his voice, a brittle edge of anger. For a moment, the energy wins us. Lenny is back. But, of course, he is not; nor is Fanny Brice or Groucho or W. C. Fields or George M. Cohan. The second-raters can be imitated; genius can only be approximated. Gorman is faced with an impossible task of impersonation. He becomes, essentially, a ventriloquist— with more talent and conviction than the policemen who recited many of Bruce's "obscene" routines for the court, but with the same task: to substitute for the genuine article. Gorman is handsome, clean-cut, conventionally literate, and has no Semitic lilt to his voice. There is nothing hard or chintzy or low-down about him. He is no "cat"; no man with an obsession. Nothing in Gorman's athletic and attractive performance conveys the emotional grit which spawned Bruce's comic pearl. Gorman is Lenny Bruce with the spiritual voltage run low, with his class toned up for the $11.50

crowd. Bruce, whose fantasies skewered the bastardization of true faith (his bit "Religions, Inc." talks of theological napkins reading: "Another Martini for Mother Cabrini."), would have something to say about the emotional rip-off of his own work. Does any revival of a comic's work debase it? Insofar as it reduces the complicated to the simple, the inventive to the trite—I think so. Lenny Bruce's life and his humor were grotesque, but not a cartoon.

I admire Tom O'Horgan, but in *Lenny* I think he has come up against a theatrical problem which his own rococo director's imagination cannot solve. Bruce was a stand-up comic, not an acrobat. The wildness of his humor was an amalgam of personality and pugnacious improvisation which bombarded an audience, with vivid, extravagant verbal images. Like the man, Bruce's laughter was lean: his rhythms were short, swift, epigrammatic. But *Lenny* is swollen with players and backdrops: the shocking becomes merely the spectacular. O'Horgan, trying to stretch the metaphor, imposes his own idea of the fantastical on Bruce's; jungle costumes (a heavy-handed and ugly symbolic incarnation of the first tribe and our primitive state), mammoth puppets (the figures of the Lone Ranger, Little Orphan Annie, Jackie "Haul Ass" Kennedy), and many other gargantuan sight gags. O'Horgan has tried to find stage images for the texture of Bruce's laughter—the peculiar burlesque broadness with which he served up some of his sharpest satire. He comes a cropper. Where Bruce acted out the voices inside his head with scrupulously accurate accents, *Lenny* divides many of the roles among the troupe, turning many of Bruce's best zingers into literal tableaux. "Christ and Moses," one of the definitive send-ups of the Church, is transformed into a vaudeville turn where the lepers actually appear, and Spellman and Sheen (unnamed for the Broadway crowd) tumble over one another with a ponderousness that would kill any joke except Bruce's best: "Sir, would you take that bell off?" Bruce bumped every joke with new surprises; O'Horgan's pacing and conception turns the unconventional into the expected. Invariably, O'Horgan makes the point with his exaggerated staging, but misses large areas of Bruce's subtlety in performance. "To Is a Preposition, Come Is a Verb" is delivered in *Lenny* like a Gene Krupa solo amid a swaying crowd, instead of the quiet, modulated interpolation it was—in which Bruce exhausted every possible combination of the words, concluding softly:

> Now, if anyone in this room or the world finds those two words decadent, obscene, immoral, amoral, asexual, the words "to come" really make you feel uncomfortable, if you think I'm rank for saying it to you, you the beholder think it's rank for listening to it, then you probably can't come. . . .

The danger (and thrill) of Bruce's performance was that of an audience confronted by a man living through his suffering in public. In the end, without an audience to hear him, Bruce talked his life minute by minute into a tape recorder. The confirmation he needed from live bodies now was left to machines. Julian Barry's book for *Lenny* creates no moment where real emotion defines or builds the foundation for genuine comic energy. Although *Lenny* ranges from 1951 to 1966, we see no progression in Bruce from Borscht-belt schlepper to authentic satirist. O'Horgan tries to mix quasinaturalistic dialogue. "Rusty"—Honey Harlow with pasties—says, "C'mon, daddy, ball me!" with his own brand of nonpsychological stage pyrotechnics. As the stage is so busy and elephantine, we can only occasionally hear Lenny's pure sound, the coruscating voice alone, brilliantly diagnosing how America's clean humor perpetuates the sickness of prejudice:

> And whatever happened to Jerry Lewis? His neorealistic impression of the Japanese male captured all the subtleties of the Japanese physiognomy. The buck-teeth malocclusion was caricatured to surrealistic proportions until the teeth matched the blades that extended from Ben-Hur's chariot. Highlighting the absence of the iris with Coke-bottle-thick lenses, this satire has added to the fanatical devotion which Japanese students have for the United States. . . .
>
> And whatever happened to Milton Berle? He brought transvestitism to championship bowling and upset a hard-core culture of dykes that control the field. From *Charley's Aunt* and *Some Like It Hot* and Milton Berle, the pervert has been taken out of Krafft-Ebing and made into a sometime-fun fag.

Society silenced Bruce. O'Horgan's final and best image —a monumental frieze of Nixon's head alongside other Presidential behemoths—makes the point. Bruce lies nude and dead on a john inside Nixon's open mouth. The sight seems even more relevant now. Censorship in the name of social health is horrific violence and a barometer of our madness. In 1970, President Nixon was maintaining:

> The warped and brutal portrayal of sex in books, plays, magazines, and movies, if not halted and reversed, could poison the wellsprings of America and Western Culture and Civilization . . . smut should not be simply contained at its present level; it should be outlawed in every state in the union.

> —*The New York Times* (October 25)

If *Lenny* capitalizes on a talent it does not serve well, Bruce's essential message is still omnipresent in the mélange of his bits. The sickness is in ourselves. His imagination reached into the recesses of American life and turned out its ugly center. Obscene, "in the classical definition of the word," is that which cannot be shown on stage *(ob scaena)*. Bruce made the word redundant. He was the first American comedian to get it all on stage. This was his lasting victory.

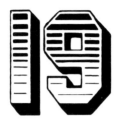

Little Richard

Little Richard always knew the power of his sound. "It's healin' music. It can make the blind see, the lame walk, the deaf and dumb hear and talk."

Rock 'n' roll kept singing that it was here to stay and no one shouted that destiny louder than Little Richard. When "Long Tall Sally" first exploded in my ears on our car radio, my father pulled off the highway and laughed for ten minutes. When Elvis, scrupulously photographed from the waist up, wiggled his way onto the Ed Sullivan Show, I fell off the sofa. Rock 'n' roll was devastating, it could paralyze you with pleasure. The music went everywhere with me. Chuck Berry for waking up; the Shirelles for whacking off; the Coasters for a late night laugh; and Little Richard for two and a half minutes of undiluted joy, any hour. Humping in the back seats of cars, studying in bed before lights out, cruising the city in a friend's set of wheels—we were sealed off in a wall of sound which was the backdrop to every personal event. And when we danced—it was still the

Lindy, then later the Swim and the Pony—we shook because, like Elvis, we felt "all shook up," because without realizing it, rock allowed us to make contact with our balls and to move at a time in the mid-1950s when all possibility for action seemed frozen. The white singers just before rock swept the country spelled their message out. I think it was Doris Day who was my nemesis. I remember trying to grab B.T. in a backseat and hearing

> Love and marriage
> Love and marriage
> Go together
> Like a horse and carriage.

They were selling a way of life, and we bought it. Or most of it. But rock 'n' roll was voodoo. It was mystery and code. You had to feel it. But if you found its secret, knew what Little Richard meant with "Wop-bop-aloo-bam-balop-bam-boom!" or how sweet the refrain "shoo-dooten-shoo-beedah" really was. It wasn't the words that stuck in the brain as much as these inarticulate syllables, sounds as full of energy and unverbalized longing as we were. And later, when the songs would play their way back through the brain, what you sang was not the words, but the high-pitched falsetto finales—of Little Willie John, Little Louis Lymon, and most especially Little Richard—a pure, impossible, almost castrated high note. That was us, jim.

Little Richard was always king. From the first moment I heard him, I knew I'd have to find him. I hunted him down in 1956 at the Loew's State. The greasers waiting on line were not like my prep-school friends. Instead of Argyle socks and white bucks, they wore leather jackets and hobnail boots. They slouched over their women, matter-of-fact about sex. I wasn't a greaser. I didn't smoke or chew. Virgin, I lived in the dream of rock's sexual promise. I ached for these motorcycle girls I'd never hang out with—these finger-popping chippies with sling-back flats and windbreakers with their names stitched—like Lester Lanin hats —over their hearts. But I was scared of their boy friends, the toughs with D.A.'s and tattoos.

There was a sense of danger in that first outing. Anything could happen when Little Richard started playing the piano. The audience was galvanized by his energy. They might take him literally and rip up the seats if he sang his song. My fantasy at the rock show was this: I'd put my arm around one of these Brooklyn vixens with pointed tits. A hood would bop over and ask if I wanted a mouthful of bloody chiclets. "My hands are registered," I'd say. The girl would lay her painted lips on mine as Little Richard howled, "Send me some lovin', send it I pray."

But it wasn't quite like that the first time. The emcee was a disc jockey who talked a mysterious argot suitable for the magical event. "Ooo-papa-doo and how are you? This is your engineer, Jocko. Saying E to the I, I to the O, let's get on with the rocketship show." The theme of the show was rockets, and no one was in a higher orbit than Little Richard. When the lights came up on him, he was even more preposterous than his voice. Dressed in an orange tuxedo, he stood with one foot on the keyboard as he caterwauled into the microphone. He sang his songs, but I'm not sure anyone heard them. The audience was singing back at him, screaming, being pulled out of their seats by cops. The important thing was to be there, to bear witness to Little Richard's flamboyance which was a kind of purity. The image of

Little Richard was indelible. He was an event, not simply a sound; something unforgettable in the forgettable normality of the time.

And now, nearly two decades later, Little Richard was back headlining a rock 'n' roll revival at Madison Square Garden's Felt Forum. Most of the performers on the bill were ghosts of themselves, as faceless as the world from which they had briefly emerged—to sing, to be famous and "on the charts," then to disappear. But not Little Richard, not yet. The famous pompadour now exaggerated into a bouffant, Little Richard pranced across the stage modeling his gaudy green-fringed costume, giving the peace sign, posing for photographs as he readied himself to pounce on the piano. Grabbing the microphone, he screamed to his audience—"Let it all hang out! It's me—Little Richard from Macon, Georgia. The man who *never* grows old."

He began the rhythmic backbeat to "Good Golly Miss Molly." The audience anticipated his squeals. "Shut up," he smiled. "I want to do it!" It was his offering, his specialty. No one could duplicate his sound, although many imitated it. He cocked his head toward the microphone. He attacked the song ferociously:

> Good golly Miss Molly
> She sure like to ball
> When you're rockin' and a rollin'
> Can't hear your Mama call

By the second chorus, the audience was filling the aisles, rushing toward the stage to dance and to be near Little Richard's energy. He was lacquered in sweat but his effort was the thrilling occasion the audience clamored for. The fans were ecstatic. Like all exciting theater, Little Richard's frenzy coaxed them out of themselves. The magic was there —that thrill of human personality radiating its essence. Janis Joplin's description of Little Richard and Tina Turner is as precise an explanation of their seismic effect on an audience as words can render. "They *work*, they *happen*, they're *electric*, they *sweat* for you. . . . You not only feel that rhythm, you not only hear it, but you see it."

Little Richard had won the audience; now he used it. He went into "Rip It Up":

> I don't care if I spend my dough
> 'Cause tonight I'm gonna be one happy soul
>
> I'm gonna rock it up
> I'm gonna rip it up
> I'm gonna shake it up . . .
> I'm gonna love it up
> And ball tonight

After a chorus, he was standing on the piano. The mob crushed close to him. He took off his beads and threw them. This surprised the audience: one woman caught the necklace without a struggle. Then his shoes: slowly, like a lubricious stripper teasing the customers, he offered up his silver slippers. The audience was a forest of waving arms. Little Richard savored the grotesque spectacle. He absorbed the power his audience surrendered to him. He toyed with the audience a few moments before throwing out his shoes. Behind him, his band, "The Crown Jewels," blared.

Now, Richard was taking off his bolero fringe top, while

a valet/bodyguard put a white towel on his shoulders. The audience swerved like pigeons waiting for crumbs. Little Richard faked throwing out his jacket. A hand reached up almost snatching it away. A moment of fear; but then Little Richard was back in control, swinging the garment to the left, then to the right. Finally, he heaved it. The jacket fell into the crowd two feet away from me. A young man clutched it tight to his chest. The magic fleece. The mob moved toward him, fighting to get a piece of the costume. Little Richard smiled with excitement at the audience. They were the real outrage, the real show, and he knew it. The young man clung to Little Richard's jacket like Ishmael to his spar. Finally, the crowd got tired of wrestling. When the audience looked back at the stage for the next song, Little Richard was gone.

A piece of green fringe from Little Richard's jacket went unnoticed on the floor as the audience filed out. I thought for a moment—of the violence, of the joy, of the pain of surviving fame, of the first time Little Richard entered my consciousness. Then I picked it up.

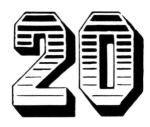

Muhammad Ali:
The Last Good-by

I sat in my seat a long time after the fight.

Joe Frazier was the first to leave the ring. He poised a split second at the edge of the steps leading down into the crowd. He shoved his hammerhead fists high into the air. There was no bravado in the gesture, just a fact. He was the winner. The Champ. Frazier, the butter-and-egg man, the man with a family of four and a rock group—The Knockouts—to back him up in his off-hour enterprises, had no illusions. Blunt, uncompromising, and as straightforward as his boxing style, he had punched his dreams into shape. This was money in the bank.

But where was the joy of victory: the ecstasy and the hope? With Frazier, the triumph was as matter-of-fact as his life. His body, his words, his personality were earthbound: he had no idea of himself except as a hard-nose puncher. Frazier was power; Ali was imagination. Perhaps that was what lured so many of us into Madison Square

Garden: the yearning to see a win that was going to be bigger than a decision; a wave of emotion which would send us higher than current events, confirming some deep, vague need to see history made decisively. There was to be something final in this fight. "This is history," someone had said, rushing to his seat. That's right, I thought. At least, in this universe of red ropes and brass boundaries, I wanted history to be clean and pure and renewing. But emotions were as stalled as the traffic in the hurly-burly of the ring. This was theater without catharsis. What had I expected?

I had wanted to be with Ali on this night, since he had been with me—somewhere in the back of my head—from my last year at Yale, when some pundit on the Yalie Daily tried to crash into his locker room after the Clay-Liston fight and talk to him about poetry. After that, I kept up with Ali. I cut out the things he said. There was something excessive and prophetic in his words. He was more than an outsider, a tragic victim, a strongman, a showboating loud-mouth: he had a pure voice, an unadulterated sound that refreshed me and sent me away from each imaginary encounter dreaming. Once planted, the seed of Ali's personality grew in me like love. It was something that could be shared. It was a common bond and an enthusiasm; an integer of speech. After all, everybody knew Ali. Sometimes I'd think how it would be if we were together: side-kicks. Ali talking in riddles, me protecting him and knowing all the time what he was saying. He'd throw a few playful jabs at my shoulder. I'd badmouth him and rock him with an uppercut to the belly. (His solar plexus would be as stiff as frozen meat.) Then we'd slap hands: the black terror and the Ivy Leaguer. "My man," he'd say. Friends. Even better than Bundini Brown. I wanted Ali to have everything: even the things I didn't want—the cars, the apartment buildings, the high times, the "foxes" hanging around to watch him skip rope or waving at him from outside his Cadillac windows. His dream was so palpable and so pained, so much deeper than that of other public figures. He wanted to be a monolith, a landmark, a spiritual leader. Ali was his own incarnation. His deeds were a testament to our faith. He was visible and elusive. Nothing from everyday life could describe his accomplishment. "Speed?" said Sonny Liston, a man who had faced the magician and was not given to poetic license. "He faster'n the wind. He kiss a bullet. He run through hell in a gasoline sportcoat and live to talk about it." Hadn't Ali himself proclaimed three months before this night, "I'm the Resurrector. The man who beats me will be remembered like the man who shot Liberty Valance." Ali carried immortality in his hip pocket. It seemed right and not too immodest to hint at such a thing. Like the other votaries, I believed; and humility from a god is as unwanted as modesty from a prostitute.

Ali watched Frazier leave. If he lost, he promised a dramatic act of humiliation typical of a saint. ("I promised Joe Frazier I would crawl across the ring on my hands and knees if he whupped me and tell him he's the greatest.") Ali had even rehearsed the gesture in training camp. He was clowning; and, like all buffoons who make pratfalls, we knew he'd bounce back. Still, the gesture seemed right for the mythic dimensions Ali created for himself. He would be as heroic in defeat as in conquest. I watched him closely with my binoculars. Bundini was crying; Ali was thinking. Slow-eyed, peaceful—Ali, I thought, was watching his career pass before him, feeling it slip away, and with it that magnetic presence we loved and longed for. But I stopped myself. That's not it. The fight's not over. Ali's going to up-stage Frazier, I kept assuring myself. His whole life had been an act of revenge, the turning of failure to outrageous success. Why not now?

"CLAY YOU STINK!" the man behind me was yelling, with no prospects of letting up.

"WHERE'S YOUR MOUTH NOW, CLAY!" Even the $160 seats were talking back after defeat. They were still afraid of that mouth: its challenge, its anger, the voraciousness behind its articulated dreams.

"YOU'RE A NOBODY, CLAY!"

The voice—beery and bone-hard—never reached the crowded ring two hundred feet below. The sound was really not so much for Ali as for the man himself. Standing in a Dacron suit with his paisley tie loosened, the man was un-fettered, screaming until the veins in his neck bulged. The man was surprised and proud of his hectoring. He was alive with rage. Even in hate, Ali was a source of energy.

No one grabbed at Frazier as his green and yellow cape bobbed amidst the crowd of police wedging its way toward the exit. But even before Ali stepped out of the ring (and despite warnings from the announcer), spectators were clutching at his body. They wanted his sweat; the magic juice of his body for good luck and strength. Their gestures were reflex; for Ali, the man who had been a transfusion of energy for America, radiated no electricity. He was listless, maybe dumbfounded. He had fired our daydreams and ap-peared in the landscape of our fantasies. We loved him for being so vivid, for acting so completely in the world: a body not shrunk behind a desk, doing part of a job, but a man whose grace, speed, and power embodied our denied freedom. In a society which wanted to make the black man invisible, Ali had fought his way not only to fortune, but to a place in the imaginative life of every American. Typical of the profound needs of the society, despite the fact that millions of people saw the battle on closed-circuit television, saw Ali's knees buckle, saw him tire, saw Frazier bludgeon him with body punches—people would still be arguing that Ali won! Days after the fight, people would ask me, "Did he really lose?"

What was puzzling was not the defeat, but the nature of Ali's performance. I had seen him firsthand once before in the Broadway production of *Big Time Buck White.* And now, while Ali tried to shake the fog out of his brain after a night's battering, staring at the crowd as his trainers rubbed his back and neck in defeat, I remembered our first meeting when he passed by close enough to touch. . . .

He entered down the aisle of the theater more solemn than tonight; his belly and arms jounced with flab, then. Ali was the fighter too smart to be hurt and too brave and proud to fight for a country that made him a champion yet enslaved his people. And yet here he was among his oppressors, walking flat-footed toward the stage in an Afro wig and fake beard. It was a sad spectacle. Ali was an imitation of himself. His first words made mockery of his stature in the ring, a destiny taken from him by the same white society now willing to pay $11.90 for the thrill of seeing him in captivity. Like Sitting Bull in Buffalo Bill's Wild West Show, Ali now owed not only his defeat, but his momentary glory to the white world. He was trapped. His first words on stage were, "I'm here to glory in my essence."

The words punished me, as they must have hurt the

blacks in the audience. "Your essence is in the ring, Ali," I said to myself. An actor accomplishes his act on the stage he chooses; and Ali's arena was that white square of canvas, elevated from the muddy brown sea of seats. Those boundaries were his liberation; the Broadway stage was clearly a jail. Like a caged bear, Ali strolled across the stage delivering his speeches and singing his songs in a soft, clear voice.

> If you think we're gonna Uncle Tom
> You might as well get your bomb
> 'Cause it's all over now, mighty Whitey
> 'Cause it's all over now. . . .

But the victory in that round was the white world's. Ali could rant at them; but he was all too clearly under control. On stage, he had no power. The spectacle boomeranged. He was not wild, nor angry, nor smart. Buck White, the fictional political hero, was all these things. Ali, the defiant victim, was simply lost. At the end of the performance, children and their mothers rushed the stage. Ali waved them away and looked down at them with avuncular reproof. His look seemed to signal that he knew this was not where he should be applauded or where he made his profoundest dreams come true. That night, at home, I wrote, "Let him finish. Let him do his thing. He is surviving. At least for the moment."

And so it grew increasingly important to see Ali on his own terrain; an actor in his own play and in his own dimension—not blown up to mammoth proportions for closed-circuit broadcasts or truncated in snapshots. But Ali—the performer—on his special stage: manipulating his world, creating a sense of himself with the timing, invention, and skill which had become legend.

The preliminaries built the drama of the main event. While the PA system buzzed Wasp organ music ("Goody-Goody for You," "Everything's Coming Up Roses"), pugs paraded into the ring to rough it up for a few rounds, their foppish colorfulness a contrast to their drab ring style. Huffing and puffing, slipping and slapping, they bashed away at one another in a crude ballet of brawn. Occasionally a fighter bobbed and weaved with a hint of excellence; but there was nothing compelling about their performances. They were nameless, faceless bodies. Theirs was just a contest of force; some of the winners even forgot to raise their hands in victory. They were the scenery against which the main event would be fought. Clumsy and uncompelling, their lack of character made the real fight even more luminous. The audience babbled about the main event and gazed through their binoculars at ringside.

"Bobby, look down there," said a girl near me to her date. "I swear that's Peter Sellers. I swear. He's gotten so thin since Britt left him."

"It says here that Ali's birth sign is Capricorn, with Leo in the ascendant," said Bobby, reading from the program. "He has a remarkable ability to summon all his energy for long-term projects or high goals and can discipline himself to achieve what he wants. He has the hunger for power and honors."

"Robert, will you look," the girl continued. Bobby keeps reading. The girl adjusts her binoculars. "That's all you think of . . . stars."

But when Ali made his entrance, the high-paying cus-

tomers found their seats. They were tense, almost prayerful
in their concern for the event. They knew more about Ali
and Frazier than they did about their own relatives. We
were all intimates of the fighters; and so the contest had become personal, the pugilists vessels of our dreams, too. Ali
was the first to enter, dressed in red and white, with jazzy
red tassels swinging arrogantly from his shoes. His costume
illustrated his vision of himself as a warrior: clean, cool, fan-
cifully above the skirmish. He was tense, but fast. He
bounced around the ring, throwing his most agile combination of jabs as Frazier stepped into the arena to great cheers.
At first, Ali paid no attention; but then, he started to
backpedal, bumping Frazier's shoulder not once but twice.
Frazier said nothing. The crowd was thrilled. Ali the show-
man was setting the stage, captivating the fans the way an
actor teases an audience with a sense of the emotional force
he's going to deliver. Even Ali's prayer, his red gloves
turned palms-up in his corner, gave this performance a
sense of mission.

Ali's abilities as an actor did not vanish with the gong for
the first round. His impersonation seemed to grow. Every
athlete talks to his opponent, egging him into mistakes; certainly, the little dramas between boxers, opposing linemen
in football, the pitcher and batter in baseball, are part of
the tension and fun of sport. But Ali's performance—even
from the beginning—was upsetting. His idea of himself as
champion, his impersonation of the undaunted warrior, was
so clear in his mind and in his actions that the fight seemed
almost an irrelevance to him. Any actor who listens to the
audience and not the rhythms and demands of his role is
hopelessly trapped between worlds. And from the beginning, this was Ali's mistake. He wasn't concentrating; and

in a play, details are everything. In the first round, talking under his white mouth guard, Ali's gestures were meant as much for the audience as Frazier. He was telling us Frazier's punches didn't hurt. He was saying in his gestures that Frazier didn't deserve to be in the same ring with him. He was showing off the mythic invincibility he had come to believe. He could not be touched by the barrage of body blows.

We had been mesmerized when Ali—then Clay—had taunted Sonny Liston, standing over him, spitting words at him, daring him to face his master. We had known that Ali could hold up a fighter, as he had Floyd Patterson, with kittenish viciousness. But his toying with Frazier was ugly and shallow. Ali shoved his long arm in Frazier's face. He pushed him off at arm's length and Frazier, as if flailing against his big brother, kept swinging in an unrelenting attempt to make contact. Ali slapped him with his glove on both sides of the face, the way a man teases a dog. At the end of the first few rounds, Ali waved his hand in disgust toward Frazier's corner. He was clowning; Frazier was trying to fight. What had gone wrong?

Ali's performance—the return he had dreamed of for so many months—had been transformed into some gruesome, self-conscious caricature. Ali seemed trapped in his own fantasy of himself, unable to see the tactical and emotional mistakes in his actions. Boxing enthusiasts may defend Ali's approach; and Ali himself may claim that in these rounds he showed clear superiority over Frazier's brute force. To me, this was of no importance. The emotional overtones of Ali's gestures, the technique which reflected the man, exposed something weak and sad in this performance. His mockery had none of the hero's courage or the warrior's resignation. He was a combatant who had lost a sense of his opponent's dignity: an actor with cast-iron instincts. Like so many stars, he seemed suddenly victim of his own press clippings; unbelieving as Frazier gradually managed to wear him down; astonished in the fourth round, when Frazier started to take control, letting down his guard and taunting Ali to come and get him. The moment was chilling. It was easy to make show. Frazier, the realist, knew he had Ali; and that no matter how theatrically Ali tried to promote his image, his capers were not enough to make victory a reality. I heard myself saying out loud, "Don't humiliate him, Joe."

Ali, the fighter cast as a national figurehead, had performed like a willful child. As a boxer, he was still strong and often impressive. He took Frazier's punishment; and despite one knockdown and a few groggy rounds where he almost toppled, he gave the fans fifteen rounds of good sport. But as a hero worthy of emulation, as an energy source, his credibility had been as badly bruised as his jaw. The resilience, the survival spirit, the concentration, and the ruthless will which lay behind the performances of the early Clay had now vanished. Ali had been cut off from the mainstream of America, only to become victim to its most stifling ethic. He wanted results without paying attention to the process. The man who had said, "I don't have to be what you want me to be. I'm free to be who I want," had fallen prey to his popularity. In the ring, it was clear Ali needed his public even more than his victory. On stage or in the boxing arena, one paradox haunted his performance: the public he defied was now strangely in control of his imagination. His freedom was an illusion.

Standing in the ring waiting to leave, Ali seemed diminished. The aura around him had evaporated. His trainer pushed a man off the steps who sprawled backward into the crowd. They were saying to make way for Ali; but it was harder now since Ali was somehow smaller.

The next day, Ali would say to the press: "It's a good feeling to lose. The people who follow you are going to lose, too. You got to set an example of how to lose. This way they can see how I lose. It'll be old news a week from now. Plane crashes, a President assassinated, a civil-rights leader assassinated. People forget in two weeks. Old news." He had spent years making a spectacle of himself, but he didn't realize the power and responsibility of his image. Was it just dumb luck? Ali still saw himself as an example. He wanted us to remember; and now he was saying we'd forget. I think he knew the truth. I did.

Walking down the ramp after the fight, a man was saying, "I'm going home and have a cry." I didn't feel emotional in the same way. I thought about Ali and me: sidekicks. I took Ali aside and cut the bandages off his fists. "Don't sweat it, Ali. Tomorrow's another day. It's a big paycheck." Ivy Leaguers know how to say the right thing.

"My main man," he said, gratefully. "See ya tomorrow?"

"Sure," I said, walking out of the dressing room, knowing this was our last good-by.

Notes

1. *Orlando Furioso:* Theater as "Contact" Sport

1. Edward T. Hall, *The Hidden Dimension* (Garden City, New York: Anchor Books, 1966), pp. 86–87.
2. Clive Barnes, "Stage: Orlando and MacGowran—Sight vs. Sense," *The New York Times* (November 27, 1970), p. 46.
3. Jacques Ellul, *The Technological Society* (New York: Vintage Books, 1967), pp. 379–80.
4. Franco Quadri, *"Orlando Furioso,"* *The Drama Review* (Vol. 4, No. 13, 1970). "A spirit of initiative, like that in popular festivals, often tempts the spectator to help actors push the floats and make himself something of a co-author, or *more* of a participant in the spectacle. This participation obviously derives from the removal of prohibitions and a return to a state of infantile immediacy . . . in the face of the fantastic and the marvelous. . . ."
5. Philip Slater, *The Pursuit of Loneliness* (Boston: Beacon Press, 1970), pp. 24–25.

2. The Theater of Sports

1. J. Huizinga, *The Waning of the Middle Ages* (New York: Doubleday and Company, 1954), p. 147.
2. Erich Auerbach, *Mimesis* (New York: Doubleday Anchor Books, 1957), p. 141.
3. C. L. Barber, *Shakespeare's Festive Comedy* (Cleveland: Meridian Books, 1963), p. 21.
4. *Ibid.*, p. 9.
5. Jacques Ellul, *The Technological Society* (New York: Vintage Books, 1967), p. 383.
6. "Radical Segregation in American Sport," by John W. Loy and Joseph F. McElvogue. From *Sport in the Socio-Cultural Process*, M. Marie Hart, editor (Dubuque: Wm. C. Brown Co., 1972), pp. 308–327.
7. *Ibid.*, p. 313.
8. *Ibid.*, p. 315.

9. *Ibid.*, p. 316.

10. Marshall McLuhan, *Understanding Media: The Extensions of Man* (New York: McGraw-Hill, 1964), p. 23.

11. Loy and McElvogue, *op. cit.*, p. 382.

12. Douglass Wallop, *Baseball: An Informal History* (New York: W. W. Norton and Company, 1969), p. 109.

13. A. Lawrence Holmes, *More Than a Game* (New York: The Macmillan Company, 1967), p. 11.

14. Jerry Kramer, *Instant Replay* (New York: World Publishing Company, 1968), p. 41.

15. *Ibid.*, p. 35.

16. Joe Namath, "I Can't Wait Until Tomorrow . . . 'Cause I Get Better Looking Every Day," *True Magazine* (September 1969), p. 54.

17. Ellul, *op. cit.*, p. 369.

18. *Ibid.*, pp. 431–32.

3. *1789:* The French Revolution Year One

The text of *1789* was published in *Gambit* (Volume 5, Number 20) and translated by Alexander Trocchi.

1. *Meyerhold on Theatre*, translated and edited by Edward Braun (New York: Hill and Wang, 1969), p. 125.

2. Interview with Ariane Mnouchkine by Irving Wardle. *Performance* (Spring 1972).

3. *Ibid.*

4. *Ibid.*

5. *Ibid.*

6. *The Memoirs of Alexander Herzen*, Vol. III (London: Chatto and Windus, 1968), p. 1236.

7. *Encounter*, "Stage Politics" (December 1971), p. 30.

8. Interview with Ariane Mnouchkine, *op. cit.*

9. *Ibid.*

10. *Ibid.*

11. *Meyerhold on Theatre*, p. 125.

12. *Ibid.*

13. Interview with Ariane Mnouchkine, *op. cit.*

4. Andre Gregory's *Alice in Wonderland:* Playing with Alice

1. Paul Weiss, *Sport: A Philosophical Inquiry* (Carbondale, Illinois: Southern Illinois University Press, 1969), p. 75.

2. J. Huizinga, *Homo Ludens* (Boston: Beacon Press, 1955), p. 48.
3. Jerzy Grotowski, *Towards a Poor Theatre* (New York: Simon and Schuster, 1969), p. 19.
4. Ralph Harper, *Nostalgia* (Cleveland: The Press of Western Reserve, 1966), p. 48.
5. Grotowski, *op. cit.*, pp. 11–18.
6. *Ibid.*, p. 16.
7. Huizinga, *op. cit.*, p. 10.
8. *Ibid.*
9. *Rat*, June 5–19, 1970, p. 4.
10. *Hard Times*, #68 (March 9–16, 1970), p. 2.
11. *Ibid.*, #81 (June 15–22, 1970), p. 1.
12. Huizinga, *op. cit.*, p. 19.

5. Pinter and Chekhov: The Bond of Naturalism

1. Quoted in David Magarshack, *Chekhov the Dramatist* (New York: Hill and Wang, 1960), p. 84.
2. *Beckett at Sixty* (London: Calder and Boyars Ltd., 1967), p. 86.
3. All Chekhov quotes are taken from: *Chekhov Plays*, translated by Elisaveta Fen (London: Penguin Books, 1954).
4. David Magarshack, *Stanislavsky: a Life* (New York: Chanticleer Press, 1937), p. 172.
5. Eric Bentley, *In Search of Theatre* (New York: Vintage Books: 1953), p. 333.
6. Magarshack, *Chekhov the Dramatist*, pp. 40–41.
7. Gore Vidal, "French Letters," *Encounter* (December 1967), p. 19.

6. Joe Orton: Artist of the Outrageous

1. R. D. Laing, *The Politics of Experience* (New York: Pantheon Books, 1967), p. 67.
2. "Joe Orton Interviewed by Giles Gordon," *Transatlantic Review*, #24, pp. 93–100.
3. Laing, *op. cit.*, p. 74.
4. *Ibid.*, p. 79.
5. *Ibid.*
6. Jason Epstein, "Bobby Seale's Trial," *New York Review of Books* (December 4, 1969), pp. 42–43.

7. Jules Feiffer and Sam Shepard: Spectacles of Disintegration

1. Robert J. Lifton, quoted in *Yale Alumni Magazine* (February 1970), p. 2.
2. Robert J. Lifton, *History and Human Survival* (New York: Random House, 1970), p. 218.
3. Lewis Chester, Godfrey Hodgson, Bruce Page, *An American Melodrama* (New York: The Viking Press, 1968), p. 520.
4. Richard Harris, *Justice* (New York: E. P. Dutton, 1970), p. 135.
5. *Ibid.*

8. Neil Simon and Woody Allen: Images of Impotence

1. Alan Harrington, *The Immortalist* (New York: Random House, 1969), p. 35.
2. R. D. Laing, *Self and Others* (London: Tavistock Publications Ltd., 1969), p. 23.
3. Quoted in Lewis Chester, Godfrey Hodgson, Bruce Page, *An American Melodrama* (New York: The Viking Press, 1968), p. 779.
4. Karl Jaspers, *Man in the Modern Age* (New York: Doubleday Anchor Books, 1957), p. 181.
5. Philip Slater, *The Pursuit of Loneliness* (Boston: Beacon Press, 1970), p. 14.

9. Mystery on Stage

1. Erich Fromm, *The Forgotten Language* (New York: Grove Press, 1957), p. 3.
2. John Russell Taylor, "Accident" *Sight and Sound* (Autumn 1966), p. 184.
3. Antonin Artaud, *Theater and Its Double* (New York: Grove Press, 1958), p. 42.
4. John Lahr, *Up Against the Fourth Wall* (New York: Grove Press, 1970), p. 173.
5. Mircea Eliade, *Myths, Dreams and Mysteries* (New York: Harper Torchbooks, 1967), p. 36.
6. Norman O. Brown, *Love's Body* (New York: Vintage Books, 1968), p. 257.
7. Jacques Ellul, *The Technological Society* (New York: Vintage Books, 1967), p. 142.
8. Eliade, *op. cit.*, p. 34.
9. *Ibid.*, p. 48.

10. Brown, *op. cit.*, p. 217.
11. R. D. Laing, *The Politics of Experience* (New York: Pantheon Books, 1967), p. 36.
12. C. G. Jung, *The Psychology of the Unconscious* (New York: Dodd, Mead, and Co., 1963), p. 36.
13. Artaud, *op. cit.*, p. 90.

10. Heathcote Williams' *AC/DC:*
Flushing the Toilet in the Brain

1. Heathcote Williams, *Gambit*, Vol. 5, #18 and 19 (London, 1972), p. 141.
2. *Ibid.*, p. 143.
3. *Ibid.*, p. 141.
4. Henry Adams, *Autobiography* (Boston: Houghton Mifflin Company, Sentry Edition, 1961), p. 381.
5. *Ibid.*, p. 499.
6. See Nicholas Johnson, "Television and Violence: Perspectives and Proposals," *Television Quarterly* (Vol. 8, No. 1).
7. *Gambit*, p. 141.
8. Bernard Rosenberg and David Manning White, *Mass Culture Revisited* (New York: Van Nostrand Reinhold Company, 1971), p. 176.
9. *Op. cit.*, p. 141.
10. *Op. cit.*, p. 176.
11. Marshall McLuhan in *Understanding Media* observes: "The aspiration of our time for wholeness, empathy, and depth awareness is a natural adjunct of electric technology. . . . The mark of our time is its revolution against imposed patterns. We are suddenly eager to have things and people declare their beings totally."
12. Harvey Cox, *The Feast of Fools* (New York: Harper Colophon Books, 1969), p. 13.
13. *Gambit*, p. 140.
14. *Ibid.*
15. *Ibid.*, pp. 140–141.
16. *Ibid.*, p. 141.
17. Gerhart Wiebe, "The Social Effects of Broadcasting," *Public Opinion Quarterly*, Vol. 33 (Winter 1969–1970).
18. H. A. Williams, *True Resurrection* (London: Mitchell Beazley, 1972), pp. 164–65.
19. Antonin Artaud, *The Theater and Its Double* (New York: Grove Press, 1958), p. 31.
20. Joseph Campbell, *Myths to Live By* (New York: The Viking Press, 1972), p. 209.

21. *Ibid.,* p. 204.
22. *Ibid.,* p. 230.
23. H. A. Williams, *op. cit.,* pp. 177–78.
24. Artaud, *op. cit.,* p. 116.

INDEX

ACKNOWLEDGMENTS

Barton Music Corp.: From "Love and Marriage," Van Huesen and Cahn. Reprinted by permission of Barton Music Corp.

The Bobbs-Merrill Company, Inc.: From *The Unseen Hand and Other Plays,* Copyright © 1972 by Sam Shepard; from *Operation Sidewinder,* Copyright © 1970 by Sam Shepard. Reprinted by permission of the publishers, The Bobbs-Merrill Company, Inc.

Wm. C. Brown Company Publishers: From *Sport in The Socio-Cultural Process* by M. Marie Hart.

Chappell & Co., Inc.: From "When I'm Not Near the Girl I Love" (*Finian's Rainbow*) © Copyright 1946 Chappell & Co., Inc.; from "Necessity" (*Finian's Rainbow*) © Copyright 1946 Chappell & Co., Inc.; from "When the Idle Poor Become the Idle Rich" (*Finian's Rainbow*) © Copyright 1947 Chappell & Co., Inc.; "One Hundred Easy Ways to Lose a Man" © Copyright 1953 by Leonard Bernstein, Adolph Green and Betty Comden. Reprinted by permission of copyright owner.

E. P. Dutton & Co., Inc.: From the book *A Theological Position* by Robert Coover. Copyright © 1970, 1971, 1972 by Robert Coover. Published by E. P. Dutton & Co., Inc. and used with their permission. "The Kid" first appeared in *Tri-Quarterly 18* (Spring 1970) .

The Harry Fox Agency, Inc.: From "Good Golly Miss Molly." Writers: John Marascalco & Robert A. Blackwell. Copyright © 1957 & 1946, Venice Music, Inc.; from "Rip It Up," Writers: John Marascalco & Robert A. Blackwell. Copyright © 1956, Venice Music, Inc.

Grove Press, Inc.: From *The Homecoming* by Harold Pinter. Copyright © 1965, 1966 by Harold Pinter Ltd.; from *What the Butler Saw* by Joe Orton. Copyright © 1969 by the Estate of Joe Orton, deceased; from *Loot* by Joe Orton. Copyright © 1967 by Joe Orton; from *The White House Murder Case* by Jules Feiffer. Copyright © 1970 by Jules Feiffer; from *The Year Boston Won the Pennant* by John Ford Noonan. Copyright © 1970 by John Ford Noonan; from *Big Time Big Buck* by Joseph D. Tuotti. Copyright © 1969 by Gard Productions, Inc.

Harcourt Brace Jovanovich, Inc.: From *Subways Are For Sleeping* by Edmund Love.

Edwin H. Morris & Company, Inc.: From "Never Never Land." From the musical production *Peter Pan.* Lyrics: Betty Comden and Adolph Green, Music: Jule Styne. © Copyright 1954 by Betty Comden, Adolph Green and Jule Styne. All rights throughout the world controlled by Edwin H. Morris & Company, Inc. Used by permission. From "Napoleon," "Leave De Atom Alone," "For Every Fish (There's a Little Bigger Fish) ," and "I Don't Think I'll End It All Today," from the Broadway musical *Jamaica,* lyrics by E. Y. Harburg, music by Harold Arlen, © Copyright 1957 by E. Y. Harburg and Harold Arlen. All rights throughout the world controlled by Harwin Music Corp.